Psychological Research Among Transgender Individuals

Harleen Kaur

Psychological Research Among Transgender Individuals

An Indian Case Study

palgrave
macmillan

Harleen Kaur
Assistant Professor
O.P. Jindal Global University
Sonipat, Haryana, India

ISBN 978-3-032-12050-2 ISBN 978-3-032-12051-9 (eBook)
https://doi.org/10.1007/978-3-032-12051-9

This Palgrave Macmillan imprint is published by the registered company Springer Nature Switzerland AG.
The registered company address is: Gewerbestrasse 11, 6330 Cham, Switzerland

Dedicated to all aspiring researchers in psychology and to the invisibly visible Indian community.

From the Author

This is an auto-ethnographic account of a researcher in psychology who is forever in the learning phase. She experimented with writing and her narrative account to bring better reading for researchers who are working for inclusive societies, especially transgender persons. The focus is solely self-identified Indian transgender persons, but this may be one of a kind where the reader feels walking along with the author and this is the only goal of the book: to make it easy for the readers. The idea is to bring forth an interactive reading tied together with academic writing. The author is open to constructive feedback and thus was able to pen whatever she was able to trace in her research journey so far, very briefly. While reading the volume remember, this is solely her interpretation of the community she is working with. She aims to be the bridge between policymakers and the community still living on the fringes of mainstream Indian society. She is a scholar advocate and she will be contained if the reader finds even one line of the volume as worthy and useful in their own journey!

It is difficult to find space when you are young! And the author is grateful for the publisher to give her that space, because whatever we say it is all the matter of space!

Acknowledgments

This auto-ethnography is the result of years of research, engagement, and personal growth, and I owe it to the many individuals and communities who shaped this journey. My deepest gratitude to the transgender community across India; your trust, stories, and resilience are the true heart of this work. A pivotal moment was my internship with the National Institute of Social Defence (NISD), Ministry of Social Justice and Empowerment, which gave me the chance to learn directly from activists and peer educators nationwide. Grateful to Dr. Veerendra Mishra, then director NISD, for motivating me to work in this field to bring me closer to this community. To Dr. Vivek Dixit, for bringing me more avenues for this community. I am indebted to my Ph.D. advisor (Prof. Singh), mentors, colleagues, and peers at Banaras Hindu University who became part of my journey. Thank you for challenging my ideas and sharpening my thinking. To my Papa, Mumma, and Janpreet, you are my grounding force. To my Husband, Sidheyndra, thank you for your patience, discipline, and belief in me. I am also grateful to activists, NGOs, and fellow researchers whose insights and solidarity made this work possible.

Special thanks to the "Pivot project," which aims to bring forth unheard voices and support young minds. To every reader, may this account not only inform but also move and inspire toward empathy and collective responsibility.

With humility and gratitude,
Harleen.

Contents

About the Author

Harleen Kaur is an assistant professor in the Jindal School of Psychology and Counselling at O. P. Jindal Global University, India. She holds a Ph.D. in Psychology from Banaras Hindu University, where her doctoral research focused on the intersectionality and lived experiences of Indian transgender persons. Her academic training also includes postgraduate qualifications in community mental health (NIMHANS), counselling, and psychological interventions. A recipient of several prestigious fellowships and international recognitions, Kaur has written widely in SCOPUS and ABDC-indexed journals and contributed chapters to volumes with reputed publishers. She serves as a peer reviewer for international journals and is the editor of a forthcoming Palgrave Macmillan volume on Global Queerness. Her expertise has also been sought in policy-level consultations with the Ministry of Health and Family Welfare, Government of India, and AIIMS on transgender healthcare. Her major areas of interest include gender and sexual minorities, cross-cultural psychology, global public health, and human rights, with a strong commitment to advancing inclusivity and mental health equity. Through her scholarship, training, and advocacy, Kaur continues to amplify marginalized voices and contribute to building culturally sensitive, socially just frameworks in psychology.

1

Introduction

Abstract This introductory chapter presents an autoethnographic account of the author's personal and academic journey into researching transgender communities in India. It explores the formative experiences and background that shaped the author's research focus, tracing a chronological path from early academic interests to a committed, community-centered approach. The narrative delves into the pivotal moments that solidified this commitment and outlines the foundational principles of building ethical, trust-based collaborations with transgender individuals. The chapter argues that meaningful research is not a detached observation but a co-created process, born from humility, reflexivity, and a genuine desire to amplify marginalized voices. It concludes with a call to action for researchers to engage in partnerships that prioritize community well-being and shared ownership of knowledge.

Keywords Researcher positionality • Autoethnography • Research ethics • Community collaboration • Transgender communities • India • Reflexivity • Trust-building • Academic journey

H. Kaur, *Psychological Research Among Transgender Individuals*,
https://doi.org/10.1007/978-3-032-12051-9_1

It wasn't a bolt of lightning that led the author here, but the gradual accumulation of softer things, the muted whispers in classrooms, the whispers recounted behind half-closed doors, the bits caught during journeys on trains through strange towns, and the echoes that were discovered in dusty, forgotten archives. These whispers formed a mosaic of fragments of lives, joys, traumas, celebrations, and silences that ultimately coalesced into the most urgent question of life back then: ***What does it mean to be transgender in India?***

This account is not born of detached academic inquiry. It is a living, breathing piece that the author feels is an amalgamation of memory, shaped by experience, and stitched together by the stories of remarkable individuals the author had the privilege of knowing. For the author, the path as a researcher was never mapped in institutional corridors or academic conferences alone. Instead, it came out of the soil of lived experience, out of the cracked sidewalks of city "bastis"/"Gharanas" (a closed knit community where Indian transgender live) and the inner spaces of community coming-togetherness, out of random meetings in waiting rooms and all-night *chai* (Indian tea) talk flavored with resistance and epiphany. This volume is the culmination of who the author was and what she has become as a researcher working with Indian transgender persons since 2019. As a researcher trained in psychology, her academic and personal journey has increasingly been shaped by a commitment to arches of social justice, inclusivity, and ethical engagement with marginalized communities. Gradually she evolved and now is working in the field of cross-cultural psychology by focusing on the human rights and health of marginalized communities.

Through the years, the author's academic inclinations have coalesced upon the lived lives of transgender persons in India. This group remains to move through systemic stigma, legal erasure, and social marginalization (Kumar et al., 2022; Meher et al., 2025).The research seeks to center transgender voices, challenge normative assumptions within psychological inquiry, and examine the intersections of identity, resilience, and agency within transgender communities. This chapter offers a reflective account of that evolving intellectual and personal journey. It provides a personal narrative of how the authors' positionality, academic training, and ethical commitments intersect with their research practice. Instead of offering facts or results, the chapter is dedicated to the frequently silent aspects of research: the incentives that attracted the author to this study, the disagreeable and ethical challenges that arose along the way, and the trans figurative collaborations that resulted from long-term contact with transgender people and collectives. In doing so, the author aims to illustrate how research is a methodological endeavor and an affective, relational, and political process shaped by the people she works with, the questions the author dares to ask, and the systems she seeks to challenge. Throughout this book Indian transgender persons are those who *self-identified* themselves.

The inception of this research journey can be traced back to the initial stages of the author's postgraduate training in psychology. In this environment, the assumed neutrality and universality of such approaches were considered uncontested to a large extent, and the author, along with many of her contemporaries, initially took these assumptions for granted without critical examination. Her education was not linear in progression but spiral, characterized by stops, digressions, and unanticipated openings. She started with questions she did not know how to pose. It wasn't until she got a chance to work very closely with the Indian transgender community that she recognized how academia could provide a vocabulary for what she already knew in my bones. Each stage of the author's' journey brought moments of awakening. Whether working with the National Institute of Social Defense (NISD), taking the Training for Augmenting Productivity and Services (TAPAS) Course, piloting research, going through a didactic community health, counseling guidance and psychological interventions, a Ph.D., or presenting papers beyond borders. But these were not always smooth climbs. There were moments of disillusionment, of wondering whether the author's' research could *truly* do justice to the lives it sought to represent.

How Has the Point of View Changed?

It happened almost serendipitously where the author was collecting data for a pilot paper of understanding perceived stress among the Indian Transgender community. The author met *Nayan* (pseudonym) at the

NISD. Nayan came there for some work; the author had almost *1 hour 23 minutes* of conversation precisely to recall. Nayan's words cracked something open inside the author. This was not theory; this was *truth*. The author saw, not just the injustice, but the *misrecognition*, a society that refused to see transgender individuals as fully human, worthy of rights, autonomy, and joy. See this for instance and think how moving the words could be?

> *Oh! so they have decriminalised us, okay? We are not criminal anymore, agree with you dear, but I have a question to ask: do they cater to us as humans?*

The author began to understand that research was not a neutral act. It was a political and ethical one. It could be extractive or it could be transformative. And she chose the latter. From that point, the author's' methodology shifted fundamentally. She began working *with* transgender communities, not *on* them. Building trust was not a step in the research process, it was its foundation. The author was very sure that the government is taking very good initiatives as she was closely reading reports, accessing resources and policies, the perk of being in NISD at that time, she was seeing how their drug de-addiction center is also taking initiatives to make transgender communities lives easy. At that phase, the conversation with Nayan struck an act of non-neutrality in the author and filled the author with an emotional being but how the author being of a scientific researcher reminded her with the act of neutrality and how it is important to strike a balance and present nothing but the truth as biasing will lead us nowhere.

Slowly, the author learned to listen before asking questions. The author offered complete transparency about the intentions, the use of data, and the outcomes. She ensured participants had veto power over how their stories were told. We developed participatory workshops where knowledge was generated together. She was constantly learning about language, about dignity, about when *not* to record. Everything was building the foundation of the author's' Ph.D. She had one principle to live by and that is to be with the truth, nothing but the truth. There were challenges, of course. Language barriers, internalized stigma, gatekeeping by institutions, and the positionality of the author as an outsider in some spaces.

But there were also triumphs. Like the time a community member said, *"You didn't just take our stories, you took the courage to speak them."*

The author first chose quantitative tools to begin researching with this community. These tools did offer insights. They promised objectivity, predictability, and generalizability. Yet, as the author slowly grew and evolved into the field, a quiet dissonance began to form with respect to this population. The author encountered moments that couldn't be neatly quantified in her understanding like the stories of their pain and resilience, expressions of identity that transcended binary categories, and cultural contexts that refused to be flattened into survey items. These moments marked the beginning of the author's' awakening and may be only then the quest to put the dissonance was set forward.

This inner conflict in her emerged during the early phase of working with transgender groups in India. Transient to conventional research, transgenderism represents a set of refined, sometimes intersectional, realities that are formed along the axes of caste, class, religion, regional identity, and the lingering legacies of colonialism. The experiences of being a transgender did not fall within the neat boxes provided by the dominant frameworks. While trying to understand, she realized that the dominant qualitative methods themselves had accidentally become complicit in obliterating the very complexities. This realization became a catalyst for a profound paradigm shift, not only in how the author went about research but, more importantly, in how she understood her role as a scholar. She started moving away from the traditional role of viewing all as an outsider toward becoming an in-loop and fully engaged participant. This shift was gradual, requiring deep unlearning and reorientation toward methodologies that honored subjectivity, narrative, and embodiment. Engaging deeply with feminist epistemologies, decolonial theory, and queer theory opened new pathways. She learned to value *situated knowledge* that is to understand that all knowing is partial, located, and relational. Participatory and ethnographic approaches became central to the authors' work, not as add-ons, but as essential to doing justice to the lives and struggles of marginalized communities. Instead of striving for objectivity through distance, she sought authenticity through proximity. There is no question about anything for quantitative research while understanding the marginalized communities but an insight that qualitative research gives a clear lens of experience through which we find themes. These themes may work as factors which we can understand with more clarity by applying either factor analysis or any other relevant statistics.

This chapter, then, is not just about the academic growth of the author, but about the ethical and emotional transformation that accompanied it. It is a story of becoming not just a better researcher but a more accountable one. Her identity as a scholar became inseparable from the author's' identity as an ally and advocate. She began to see research not merely as a means of knowledge production, but as a tool for social change. Interwoven with this journey are intimate reflections on identity and belonging, both of her's and those of the communities she works with. The boundaries between the personal and empathetic, the academic and the activist, began to unfurl and that gave the understanding to listen more deeply, to embrace ambiguity, and to be guided by the principle of *doing no harm* while striving to *do good.* Soon the author was no longer interested in speaking *about* transgender lives; she sought to collaborate, co-create, and speak *with* and *alongside.* To be comprehensive, the author's' trajectory as a researcher who sought interest in social policy has been one of disruption and realignment, from statistical abstraction to embodied solidarity. From a position of theoretical detachment to one of ethical entanglement. The academia taught her to ask questions; the field taught her to be a listener. This chapter is both a reflection and a commitment, to continually keep a quest for learning, from experimenting from methods, to remain accountable to the communities I work with, and to foreground the voices that dominant paradigms often silence.

Early Academic Background and Foundational Experiences in Psychology

The author's' academic formation was grounded in the empirical rigor of social psychology, which she believes is a discipline where the elegance of numerical precision and the realities of statistical modeling offered powerful tools to dissect and understand human behavior. During these formative years, one could say my mind was captured by phenomena such as group dynamics, intergroup relations, and identity-authorization being boiled down into variables, then these variables being connected through correlations and finally interpreted in terms of predictive models. As such, standardized surveys and psychometric scales would stand out in the methodology: they provided for an apparent objectivity and replicability which were appealing to scientists wishing to identify universal truths.

However, an element of dissonance began to emerge even in these initial forays. The author became increasingly aware of how limiting the quantification of the human experience was, particularly when used upon populations whose realities were difficult to pin down in concrete terms. Matters at the border attracted my intellectual attention: social exclusion, struggles over identity, and systemic invisibilization of minority voices. It was at this point that her early attraction to numbers met an intellectual and ethical impasse. She had come to see that for communities subjected to a long history of epistemic erasure, such as transgender persons in India, the very standard instruments themselves failed to locate affective, lived experiences. She pens her narrative in the following chapters as to how this realization came into my being. This curiosity deepened as I engaged more seriously with the lived realities of transgender communities in India, where the interplay of caste, gender nonconformity, and cultural tradition creates a highly complex matrix of marginality. In the literature she came across, especially concerning the psychosocial aspects of transgender identity, there existed a blatant contrast. On the one hand, social psychologists would have offered a framework to measure disparities in access to, say, education or healthcare or employment. Conversely, ethnographic narratives and narrative-driven studies illuminated the affective implications of estrangement from family, the vulnerability of makeshift dwelling, the politics of visibility among hijra groups, and the multi-level trauma of navigating public space. Through these readings and experiences, my scholarly thinking was reconfigured. The author began to understand that while quantitative approaches could powerfully demonstrate the *extent* of inequality, they were often silent on the texture of lived experience. Gradually she started realizing that statistical models could outline the frequency of discrimination but could not translate the emotional labor required to survive it. Pain, resilience, and resistance integral to understanding marginalized identities resist clean numerical encapsulation. This recognition fueled a growing commitment to integrating qualitative methodologies, particularly narrative inquiry, phenomenology, and may be participatory research, into my work. It became apparent that to learn about the communities she intended to represent, she required a wider methodological vision, one that could contain complexity without reducing it to simplistic categories. In the hindsight, this time was not only a methodological adjustment but a political awakening. It was making that author attuned to the politics of knowledge-making, compelling her to wonder whose voices were being called upon and whose voices were being erased in the academic record. It was from this perspective that she began reading about transgender studies in India not only as a research object, but as a space of decolonial resistance, epistemic experimentation, and radical care.

Methodologies and Their Limitations

A turning point in her research journey was when she first tried to gather survey data from a group of transgender individuals in western India. Then, she was still working in the prevailing paradigms of social psychology based on the belief that standardized measures like the highly applied Perceived Stress Scale (PSS) would provide objective and generalizable knowledge about the experience of marginalized groups. The author vividly remembers administering the PSS to a group of forty transgender participants, all from the same local community. What she expected to be an individual, introspective exercise in rating stress levels quickly became something else entirely. As the participants gathered, they began discussing the questions among themselves quite openly. *"It was very easy,"* one of them said cheerfully. *"We asked each other what to fill and we filled the same."* The author was startled to discover that all forty individuals had marked nearly identical responses across each item on the scale. What was intended to be forty distinct data points, forty windows into individual experiences, had, in practice, produced only one. Still committed to the "scientific process" she tried again the following day; this time requesting that they complete a different psychological test in her presence, in silence, to ensure individual reflection. But the outcome was remarkably similar. Despite her efforts to control for peer influence, participants once again consulted with one another and answered uniformly. The gesture was not one of rebellion but of community. Their reaction was one of collective consciousness, of shared resilience and solidarity forged out of years of having negotiated stigma and survived as a group. Pain wasn't internalized; decisions weren't made in solitude in their world. The very logic of psychometric measurement so heavily predicated on individualism stood in stark contrast to the communal ways of being and knowing that characterized this group.

This experience was a profound revelation. On paper, the author had attempted to produce clean, quantifiable data from forty individuals. In reality, she was only one shared narrative repeated forty times. Statistically, it was being treated sincerely as $n = 1$ sample. It was humbling to consider it seriously. It now appeared that the quantitative methods were not only secondary and would possibly deceive under those circumstances where the pacts for common survival and communal identity govern individual experiences. Moreover, she was forced to reckon with the practical limitations of her research design. In order to derive statistically valid results using psychometric tools, she would have needed a much larger sample, at least 300 individual responses to ensure the robustness required later *(if she was to develop this pilot into my thesis)*. Given the challenges of recruitment, trust-building, and ethical engagement within this marginalized community, such a number was impossible for a single researcher to achieve in their doctoral reserach. This became best of her understanding.

This was the moment when the author decisively reoriented her methodological approach. Instead of starting out with quantification, she opted to immerse herself qualitatively beforehand, through interviewing, narrative, and participant observation. This enabled the author to engage richly with the stories, feelings, and cultural reasoning that constitute transgender lives in India. Instead of starting out with quantification, she opted to immerse herself qualitatively beforehand, through interviewing, narrative, and participant observation. This enabled her to engage richly with the stories, feelings, and cultural reasoning that constitute transgender lives in India. Only after understanding the community's collective language of experience did she consider developing or adapting quantitative instruments that might resonate more authentically. She was still going back and forth with the data she had collected in her internship and my doctoral. She uses a different qualitative analysis to understand their narratives better.

Interaction with Transgender Realities

The author's transformation as a researcher was not born solely in academic texts or university classrooms, but in the immersive and often emotionally charged spaces of community engagement. A very crucial turn that her research aptitude took was during her internship with the NISD, where she had the opportunity to participate in the Training of Trainers on "Drug Abuse Prevention for Peer Educators of the Transgender Community" held on February 19–20, 2020 (Fig. 1.1). The two-day workshop by the Social Defence Division brought together transgender activists and peer educators from across India. It wasn't just training, it became a space of reflective exercises, networking, and honest sharing, where stories of vulnerability, substance use, and systemic neglect were voiced with such openness that they left a lasting impact on the author (NISD, 2020). The program acknowledged a crucial reality: the transgender community in India is among the socioeconomically marginalized, and this marginalization often intersects with substance use and abuse, exacerbated by exclusion from families, schools, employment, and healthcare. She still remembers a session where a peer educator spoke about how internalized stigma pushes many transgender individuals toward substance use, not just as an escape but as a way to cope with years of rejection. What stayed with her was not only the weight of these struggles but the incredible strength with which people turned their pain into advocacy becoming pillars of support in their own communities.

As an intern, the author was positioned at the crossroads of observation and participation. The stories shared during the sessions and the dynamic, culturally grounded ways in which peer educators approached harm reduction opened her eyes to the disjuncture between textbook interventions and community-rooted realities. The experience reinforced

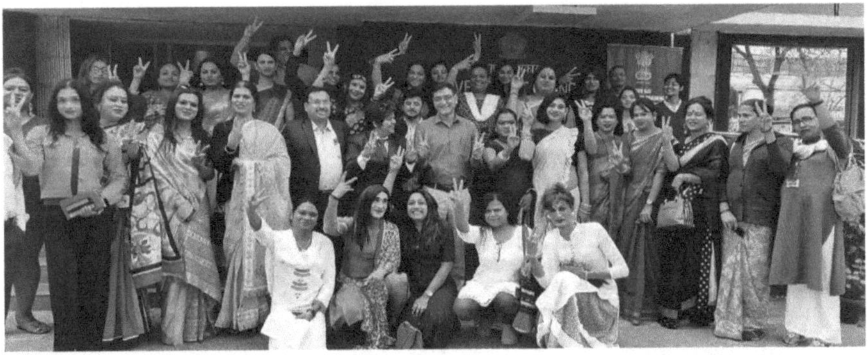

Participants at the two-day national-level "training of trainers" programm. on Drug Abuse Prevention for Peer

Fig. 1.1 Participants at the two-day national-level "training of trainers" programm. on Drug Abuse Prevention for Peer. (Source: NISD Annual Report 2019–2020. https://www.nisd.gov.in/annual_report/annual_report19-20.pdf)

a truth she was already beginning to understand that real change cannot be created from a distance.

This program along with her earlier field experiences became a turning point for reflection and change in how she approached her work. She started to see the role of a researcher not as an outsider taking knowledge but as a learner walking alongside others in a shared effort for social change. She kept asking herself how can research truly honor the stories she hears. How can she make sure that the realities of gender trauma survival and substance use are not flattened into mere data or labels *(etic vs. emic approaches as we understand)*.

It was in this context that the author firmly committed to a participatory and qualitative research approach. The narratives she encountered both during this NISD training and in other community settings made it clear that traditional tools, no matter how scientifically validated, could not fully hold the emotional and cultural depth of transgender lived experiences. She recognized the need to first center these voices through open-ended dialogues and life stories, and only then consider quantitative strategies for triangulation or broader generalization. In retrospect, the NISD program was a bridge; to the author it was connecting her academic training with grassroots realities, linking data with dignity. It showed her that empathy, ethical responsibility, and humility are not just values but essentials when working with marginalized communities, and it was here that she began to see research not only as producing knowledge but as listening, learning, and standing in solidarity.

Understanding the Complexities of Transgender Lived Experiences

At the heart of this journey was the realization that transgender lives in India cannot be understood only through gender or identity; they are also shaped by caste, class, religion, and local cultural practices. Studies have shown that these intersections deepen exclusion while also shaping the ways transgender people find and live their identities. There is sufficient literature to support that the author deeply was on hijra communities which revealed how transgender identities in India are rooted in cultural history rituals and social life (Kalra, 2012; Mal, 2018; Mondal et al., 2020; Roy, 2016). The hijra community with its traditions, networks and collective identity challenged the narrow binary models from the "West" and showed the author that identity here is not just medical or psychological but also profoundly cultural and social (Bhattacharya & Ghosh, 2020; Billard & Nesfield, 2020). This holistic perspective was a turning point in her research philosophy, prompting her to adopt an intersectional framework that places lived experiences at the center of inquiry. Moreover, participatory research models allowed her to appreciate the dialectical relationships between the individual and society (Cornwall & Jewkes, 1995; Petras & Porpora, 1993; Schubotz, 2019; Van der Riet, 2008; Wallerstein & Duran, 2017). For instance, the narratives of discrimination and economic marginalization as discussed in several seminal works underscored how systemic structures of power shape mental health outcomes and everyday lived realities for transgender individuals (Gerwe, 2025; Hermaszewska et al., 2022; Hui et al., 2021; Lacombe-Duncan et al., 2022; Suleman et al., 2024; Wesp et al., 2019).

To understand the complexities of transgender lives, one needs to understand first who is a transgender and just after that one would be curious to know who is an Indian transgender? The next chapter will closely make one understand what is the reality of a transgender in India through authors' understanding. She realized the need to break down these power dynamics as she went through archives of ethnographic studies and community testimonies that revealed the many ways stigma, violence, and exclusion shape everyday life.

References

Bhattacharya, S., & Ghosh, D. (2020). Studying physical and mental health status among hijra, kothi and transgender community in Kolkata, India. *Social Science & Medicine, 265*, 113412.

Billard, T. J., & Nesfield, S. (2020). (Re) making "transgender" identities in global media and popular culture. In *Trans lives in a globalizing world* (pp. 66–89). Routledge.

Cornwall, A., & Jewkes, R. (1995). What is participatory research? *Social Science & Medicine, 41*(12), 1667–1676.

Gerwe, C. (2025). Navigating the complexities in gender-diverse counseling: Understanding the interplay of gender identity, racial inequities, economic marginalization, and aging. *Journal of LGBTQ Issues in Counseling, 19*(3), 286–301.

Hermaszewska, S., Sweeney, A., Camminga, B., Botelle, R., Elliott, K., & Sin, J. (2022). Lived experiences of transgender forced migrants and their mental health outcomes: Systematic review and meta-ethnography. *BJPsych Open, 8*(3), e91.

Hui, A., Rennick-Egglestone, S., Franklin, D., Walcott, R., Llewellyn-Beardsley, J., Ng, F., et al. (2021). Institutional injustice: Implications for system transformation emerging from the mental health recovery narratives of people experiencing marginalisation. *Plos One, 16*(4), e0250367.

Kalra, G. (2012). Hijras: The unique transgender culture of India. *International Journal of Culture and Mental Health, 5*(2), 121–126.

Kumar, G., Suguna, A., Suryawanshi, D. M., Surekha, A., Rajaseharan, D., & Gunasekaran, K. (2022, November). Exploring the discrimination and stigma faced by transgender in Chennai city-A community-based qualitative study. *International Journal of Family Medicine and Primary Care, 11*(11): 7060–7063. https://doi.org/10.4103/jfmpc.jfmpc_1037_22. Epub 2022 Dec 16. PMID: 36993073; PMCID: PMC10041271

Lacombe-Duncan, A., Jadwin-Cakmak, L., Trammell, R., Burks, C., Rivera, B., Reyes, L., et al. (2022). "… Everybody Else Is More Privileged. Then It's Us…": A Qualitative study exploring community responses to social determinants of health inequities and intersectional exclusion among trans women of color in Detroit, Michigan. *Sexuality Research and Social Policy, 19*(4), 1419–1439.

Mal, S. (2018). The hijras of India: A marginal community with paradox sexual identity. *Indian Journal of Social Psychiatry, 34*(1), 79–85.

Mondal, B., Das, S., Ray, D., & Banerjee, D. (2020). "Their Untold Stories…": Lived experiences of being a transgender (Hijra), A qualitative study from India. *Journal of Psychosexual Health, 2*(2), 165–173.

Meher, B., Acharya, A. K., & Pallotta-Chiarolli, M. (2025). Transgender women in India: Neocolonialism, stigmatization and discrimination. *Journal of Homosexuality, 72*(10), 2056–2073.

NISD. (2020). Annual Report 2019–2020. https://www.nisd.gov.in/annual_report/annual_report19-20.pdf, p. 34.

Petras, E. M., & Porpora, D. V. (1993). Participatory research: Three models and an analysis. *The American Sociologist, 24*(1), 107–126.

Roy, J. (2016). Translating hijra into transgender: Performance and pehchān in India's trans-hijra communities. *Transgender Studies Quarterly, 3*(3–4), 412–432.

Schubotz, D. (2019). *Participatory research: Why and how to involve people in research*. Sage.

TAPAS. (2025). https://tapas.dosje.gov.in/

Suleman, D., Kashif, A., Gul, S., Hamid, S., & Yunus, A. (2024). Navigating shadows: The impact of social stigma on the mental health of the transgender community in South Asia. *Migration Letters, 21*(1), 167–181.

Van der Riet, M. (2008). Participatory research and the philosophy of social science: Beyond the moral imperative. *Qualitative Inquiry, 14*(4), 546–565.

Wallerstein, N., & Duran, B. (2017). The theoretical, historical and practice roots of CBPR. *Community-based Participatory Research for Health: Advancing Social and Health Equity, 2*, 25–46.

Wesp, L. M., Malcoe, L. H., Elliott, A., & Poteat, T. (2019). Intersectionality research for transgender health justice: A theory-driven conceptual framework for structural analysis of transgender health inequities. *Transgender Health, 4*(1), 287–296.

2

Understanding Indian Transgender Realities

Abstract This chapter challenges monolithic portrayals of transgender individuals in India by employing an intersectional lens to examine the complexities of their identities. It argues that experiences of gender are profoundly shaped by interlocking factors of caste, class, religion, region, and socioeconomic background, creating unique landscapes of both marginalization and resilience. The chapter provides a historical overview of transgender communities, connecting past cultural contexts to present-day social, political, and economic realities. By highlighting diverse narratives and lived experiences, it moves beyond a homogenized view to reveal a vibrant mosaic of identities. The analysis underscores that effective advocacy and support must be nuanced and responsive to this intricate tapestry of intersecting lives.

Keywords Intersectionality • Identity • Caste • Religion • Socioeconomic status • Hijra • Historical context • Discrimination • Resilience • Diversity

H. Kaur, *Psychological Research Among Transgender Individuals*,
https://doi.org/10.1007/978-3-032-12051-9_2

In Chap. 1, the journey of the author is described from viewing the topic mainly through academic concepts and frameworks to developing genuine empathy and insight into the lived realities of transgender individuals. Soon the author recognized the limits of staying on the outside as an observer and stressed the importance of understanding transgender lives directly through the voices of those who experience them. This chapter is penned to widen the lens of the curious minds, diving into the rich collection of identity as it exists within transgender communities in India. Here, we'll explore how intersecting factors, gender, caste, religion, socioeconomic background combine to form unique identities. It is different from the one-dimensional portrayals by acknowledging a spectrum of diverse, lived experiences. By examining historical legacies, contemporary challenges, and ongoing movements, one can start to grasp the dynamic, resilient nature of transgender lives in India today. The understanding should begin with getting a conceptualisation of how law in the Indian diaspora unfurls for transgender persons (Clark et al., 2025).

How Is It to Live as an Indian transgender Person as per Law?

Section 377 was introduced to decriminalize same-sex acts and eminent persons called this legislation discriminatory of the LGBTQ+ community (Baudh, 2013; Gupta, 2006). This section was enacted by the British in the nineteenth century to prohibit "carnal intercourse against the order of nature," chiefly to prevent sexual practices that were against Victorian moral codes (Bhaskaran, 2013; Soohinda et al., 2025). This colonial law became the chief stigma between the institutional, social, and legal mechanisms that continually oppressed sexual minorities, while also evolving an unfair binary conception of gender and sexuality that disadvantaged several indigenous Indian communities. Although the honorable Supreme Court of India reinterpreted Section 377 and ended the prosecution of private consensual sexual conduct among adults in the now-famous Navtej Singh Johar case, the Court did not strike down the statute (Soohinda et al., 2025). Among its purposes, the Transgender Persons

(Protection of Rights) Act 2019 aimed at granting legal and statutory protections to transgender persons, apart from the judicial activism like in the NALSA judgment, which recognized transgender persons as "third gender" starting from 2014 (Bhattacharya et al., 2022; Hossain, 2017; Jain et al., 2025). The full fulfillment of human rights and the elimination of discriminatory practices that were put in place during colonial rule are hampered by the persistence of colonial legal frameworks in both language and practice, even in the face of these reforms.

The feud between residual colonial ideals and progressive jurisprudence finds a compellingly convincing illustration in the evolution of the legal reforms in India. A break was made in 2009 with a ruling of the Delhi High Court implementing a first challenge to Section 377 while emphasizing the rights of privacy and human dignity, thus breaking away from an otherwise restrictive legal tradition. Unable to bear this setback, the intense agitation of courts and public opinion ultimately culminated in the 2013 honorable Supreme Court verdict which restored to it a brief unfortunate period of oppression (Jain et al., 2025; Singh et al., 2022). Legal amendments undertaken in isolation without interfacing adequately with the prevailing social ethos tend to be rather frail, a weakness clearly reflected during this period in the oscillation of legal interpretations between the liberal and the conservative.

Transgender Persons (Protection of Rights) Act, 2019

The Act came into existence purely to protect transgender people from discrimination in various spheres, including the workplace, healthcare, educational setup, and so on (Balabantaray & Singh, 2022; Chandra, 2017; Saraff et al., 2022). But on closer scrutiny, it may be observed that the Act has substantive as well as procedural lacunae, which undermine the intended revolutionary effect of its enactment (Singh et al., 2023). One of the major criticisms against the Act is that it requires all transgender people to procure a gender identity certificate from the District-Level Screening Committee. Not only is this a cumbersome and invasive process, but it is also a way of reinstating state control over personal autonomy (Ata et al., 2025).The mechanism sustains the historically bad idea that transgender bodies are abnormal in one way or the other and, therefore, must be regulated, thus limiting the agency of others instead of furthering the empowerment of transgender persons. More criticisms of this law emphasize its tokenistic character because a minimal degree of recognition is given to a person under the law, lacking the substance of implementation for some meaningful improvement. For instance, even while the Act specifically prohibits discrimination in various fields, there is no reference to any enforcement or sanction mechanism to be followed in cases of default (Waggy & Bashir, 2025). Further, the Act tends to overlook or deliberately discount the problems of other groups, such as transgender men and non-binary persons, in favor of the demands and experiences of trans women and hijras. The categories of persons rarely hold a colloquy of selective legal inclusions that juridically value some transgender identities over others, resulting in uneven infusions of rights and protections foregrounding social and institutional neglect (Bhattacharya et al., 2022; Mehta, 2021). Lastly, there is much more occurring under the implementation mantle; these immensely dilate the ills of the Act. Inconsistent access to the rights and services that the "Act" ostensibly guarantees has been caused by the discretionary power of government authorities in processing identity documents, pervasive disinformation, and a lack of sensitivity training among service providers. This is what can be seen in the fields of education and healthcare where transgender persons are still a minority because there are heteronormative attitudes in society and there are traditional institutional practices ongoing (Balabantaray & Singh, 2022). So, it is safe to say that despite the Act is progressive in nature, but to a larger extent it ignored the systemic causes of inequality and exclusion (Chandra, 2017; Jain, 2022; Saraff et al., 2022).

Understanding Intersectionality

The recurrent theme noticed in literature is of elite financiers of LGBTQ+ rights obscuring the issues of the marginalized, including Dalit, Adivasi, and working-class trans people (Das, 2025; Mukherjee, 2023). This keeps intact hierarchized narratives within the queer movement. There are two necessities in India's activism: the mass movement centered on socioeconomic grievances and exclusions based on caste, and the second one centered on gaining official legitimation in the form of judicial and legislative progress. The very symbolic reduction of Section 377 to represent homophobia has been contested by activists who argued that this focus silences the voices of individuals confronting myriad forms of marginalization while raising high on the list of loudspeakers the very limited experiences of an elite class (Srivastava & Kumar, 2019). Although the Transgender Persons Act is a sign of progress, it also draws attention to conflicts between the needs of transgender populations, especially those in low-income and rural areas, and symbolic legal achievements. Certainly working passionately in the field, hearing the tales of self-identified persons, and going through the literature, the author believes that an intersectional framework that actively addresses the structural causes of inequality is required in India (Crenshaw, 1991). Not only that, advocating for legalization and rights recognition is essential for future action for all stakeholders (Mehta, 2021). Such activism should build solid networks that combine legal lobbying with actual community support so that changes are not merely verbal victories but rather real agents of change in the world. Refocusing activist strategies would allow its tenants to critically engage state institutions to support changes in social service delivery, policing procedures, and public policy that take into account the multitude of experiences of queer and trans people. Community consultations and participatory research methods help reduce bias in policy-making and make sure underrepresented voices are included in both shaping and implementing reforms (Opia, & Matthew, 2025). This can move the movement to remove the last vestiges of colonial legal philosophy and make way for an all-encompassing emancipation that includes both institutional and cultural transformation through intersectionality as a framework in both legal critiques and activist means.

A crucial transformation in this research journey was the growing recognition that the lives of transgender individuals in India cannot be meaningfully understood through the isolated lens of gender identity alone as mentioned before in the introduction. Rather, their experiences are deeply enmeshed within a broader matrix of social determinants such as caste, class, religion, regional history, and cultural tradition, that co-construct and often compound the nature of their marginalization (Boskey, 2014). In this understanding any attempt to engage with transgender realities without attending to these interlocking axes of identity would be not only analytically insufficient but ethically irresponsible. This understanding of intersectionality formed the conceptual and methodological foundation of the doctoral research pursued later. This book grew out of both academic work and close field experiences, which showed the urgent need to see transgender identities not as deviations from the norm, but as rich, lived realities shaped by overlapping systems of oppression and resilience.

The author's immersion in intersectional scholarship, particularly within the Indian context, was instrumental in shaping this approach. Seminal work, such as by Kalra, attempted to make us understand how hijra communities possess culturally anchored gender identities beyond the "'Western"' binary system (Kalra, 2012). Such identities are not merely individual experiences of gender dysphoria but are embedded in traditions, community rituals, and socio-religious roles. This perspective helped the author move past the limits of Eurocentric models that often medicalize or pathologize transgender identities, and instead see them as relational, historical, and socially grounded. Further, participatory and narrative-based research approaches allowed her to explore how transgender subjectivities are negotiated at the intersection of systemic structures and personal agency. Pinna and her colleagues in 2022 put forth an insightful systematic review that was critical in highlighting how caste-based exclusion and economic marginalization profoundly impact mental health outcomes for transgender individuals (Bhattacharya & Ghosh, 2020; Singh et al., 2025). Slowly through working more toward this population, the author came across various accounts demonstrating how structural violence operates not just in obvious discrimination, but also in chronic precarity like the denial of access to stable shelters, education, health, and work.

The intersectional framework proved essential as she engaged with the lived realities of transgender women coming from different socioeconomic statuses, geographical dividend, age whose experiences of gender-based stigma were intensified by caste hierarchies. Their voices disrupted any single narrative of trans identity and insisted on a more complex perspective, one that would track how oppression compounds across social systems. The histories were able to retract from the available literature and archival research uncovered additional layers of complexity, including how regional traditions, religious identities, and generational trauma structured individual identity formations and resistance strategies. Throughout the course of her doctoral research, intersectionality was more than a conceptual framework; it was a methodological allegiance aligning with political position. In situating lived experience at the forefront of her research she engaged with participants not as data but as epistemic actors. She believed this is crucial for knowledge construction (Ben-ari & Enosh, 2011; Kaur & Singh, 2024; Pandya & Radcay, 2021).

The Interpretative Phenomenological Analysis (IPA) approach was used to allow this depth to occur, permitting reflexivity, co-construction of meanings, and emotional attunement to the lifeworlds of the participants (Nizza et al., 2021; Smith, 2011, 2017). The research established that lives of the transgender persons in India are lived at the tangled intersections of multiple categories of social identity. To look upon these lives responsibly is to respect that complexity, not to flatten it into mere variables, but to understand it by way of rich, contextual, and collaborative research praxis. This commitment to intersectionality marks her from the dissertation days and serves as the very benchmark through which she gauges all subsequent scholarship, advocacy, and methodology.

Transitioning from Detached Observation to Engaged Scholarship

The path from observer to engaged and empathetic scholar was gradual and sometimes humbling. The author had to release worn assumptions of objectivity, of neutrality and of researcher/researched binary. This process was facilitated by difficult questions, occasions of uncertainty, and ethical dilemmas and by a growing realization that conventional research could never possibly contain the richness and nuance of transgender lives in India. In earlier training as a social psychologist, one is taught to maintain analytical distance, to minimize "bias," and to rely on standardized tools to ensure replicability and generalizability. While such tools had their place, especially in controlled settings, they were sometimes not beneficial for the aim of studying these populations when their lived experiences are at the center. As the author began working with marginalized transgender individuals whose lives unfolded within layers of structural violence, community resilience, and cultural specificity, she realized the quest of qualitative lenses. In her understanding, the categories of conventional research, stress scores, satisfaction indices, symptomatology, could not contain the emotional, spiritual, and social breadth of their experiences completely. This realization marked a turning point in the author's academic inquiry; she came to understand that she must be inseparable from social responsibility. It is not enough to study marginalized communities; one must stand with them. Influential advocacy-oriented studies in transgender health and rights, particularly those that emphasized *participatory ethics and knowledge co-production* helped her recognize the potential of research not just to describe but to intervene meaningfully (Page, 2022). From this point forward, she consciously shifted her orientation from research *on* communities to research *with* communities. The Government changed into an active participant in a community transformation process through the methodological change to Community-Based Participatory Research (CBPR). CBPR considered participants collaborators that set research questions, designed instrument measures, interpreted results, and set the methods of dissemination—for example, in contrast to other forms of social research where subjects were passive data sources. This model not only challenges conventional hierarchies of knowledge but also ensures that the research process remains embedded in local needs, wisdom, and aspirations (Wallerstein & Duran, 2006). Older theories of identity in psychology have often drawn on fixed, prescriptive models that struggled to integrate the flowing, intersectional concepts of gender seen in transgender lives (Hauge, 2007). By contrast, continued immersion in community storytelling has pointed to the dynamic, unfolding process of identity as it is continuously remolded and reshaped by individual experiences, cultural norms, and structural forces (Collins, et al., 2018).

Historically, one needed to sit with transgender elder members or community leaders, opening one's ears to the utmost attention, as these esteemed figures debated among themselves about what questions should be asked and how. That is, their epistemologies, agendas, and cultural practices were allowed to shape the design and tempo of one's learning. In these conversations, one is not an expert but is a guest, a willing learner, and a collaborator. Rather than an extraction of knowledge, the research functioned as a dialogue in which knowledge could be drawn forth more deeply, in richer ways, and on more solid ground from within the perspective of those who lived the reality. Having made this methodological shift, the researcher also had to engage in moral accountability. Participatory research is not just about changing who participates; it is about reimagining what an ethical engagement looks like. The researcher becomes more and more aware of how traditional research relationships are fraught with imbalances of power: who asks questions, who owns and controls the data, who gets cited, and who never sees their names in print. These reflections led one to develop research protocols based on trust, reciprocal exchange, and joint authorship. Slowly one is committed to instituting community feedback loops, assured data sovereignty, and consent practices.

One of the most radical elements of this ethical shift was seeing research itself as a potential tool of empowerment. As transgender people co-analyzed their own stories, they not only took back their tales from academic abstraction but also discovered patterns, strengths, and modes of resistance. The process of analysis frequently had therapeutic and political implications, enabling participants to envision themselves as producers of knowledge, rather than objects of research. The author also became deeply aware of how exclusionary practices even in well-intentioned research can replicate the very silencing they seek to expose. For example, traditional language in surveys and interviews often failed to capture the complexity of local gender categories or modes of expression. CBPR pushes one to recraft their tools and measures, in concert with community participants, so that they were not only culturally competent linguistically but also culturally resonant (Collins et al., 2018). Through such collaborative tuning, both the parties that are the researcher and the participants can craft questions and structures that respect the multiple vocabularies and worldviews of Indian transgender communities.

The journey into engaged scholarship changed what doing research means to a researcher. It became about letting go, stepping into discomfort and valuing humility more than certainty. It taught the author that curiosity should be an act of solidarity, one that empowers rather than objectifies, one that listens patiently before it speaks. It is this ethos of participatory, accountable, and ethically grounded research that now guides her work across all domains which are academic, activist, and pedagogical in nature. Research on mental health in elderly transgender communities and on socioeconomic exclusion in rural versus urban settings further influenced pursuing these intersecting axes through participatory and narrative methods (Page et al., 2016). This further reinforced the author's belief that transgender studies research needs to be holistic, extensively contextual, and committed to social justice.

Methodological Learnings

Being based on quantitative methods that involve pre-validated scales and statistical analyses in the best of authors' understanding such methods have thin success in capturing the fluid, nuanced, and culturally specific dimensions of transgender identity in India. For example, while standardized tools can measure things like gender dysphoria or psychological distress, they often miss the everyday social pressures that transgender people face because of systemic discrimination and cultural marginalization. This limitation gave the author methodological understanding where she incorporated qualitative measures of in-depth interviews, focus groups, and narrative analyses into her research designs. Through these qualitative approaches, she was able to capture the idiosyncratic, everyday realities of transgender people, stories of resilience in the face of adversity, accounts of familial rejection and forced marginalization, and narratives that illustrated the profound impact of social stigma on mental health. One study she encountered which detailed the lived experiences of transgender women and hijra in Vadodara, highlighted how cultural traditions, collective community practices, and hierarchical structures, such as those within the hijra gharana, shaped identity and coping strategies (Mazumdar, 2016). Such insights compelled the author to adopt a mixed-methods approach that offered both breadth and depth, allowing for a more comprehensive understanding of the complexities revolving around transgender voices (Arvind et al., 2022).

Moreover, these qualitative methodologies were instrumental in unveiling the intersectional nature of oppression. Research began to interrogate how overlapping identities, such as those influenced by caste, class, regional culture, and even age, interacted to compound the vulnerabilities faced by transgender individuals. The shift that happened in the research was not merely an academic one but one with very important personal connotations. The more she worked with transgender communities in interviews, workshops, and participatory sessions, the further she saw her job beyond mere professional inquiry. It was an enlightening experience, telling that research is not only about understanding society but also about fomenting change and advocating for it. But while conversing, she would watch that stigma and exclusion like a trap being released and then falling onto human minds and spirits. Stories of rejection by family, of financial crises, and of the debilitating daily toll of microaggressions poured in alongside affirmations of our strength, hope, and fight for dignity and recognition.

> *Where you live matters. When you fall sick it is better understood that one should live near such facilities but not everyone can afford good localities with hospitals. I remember I accidently cut my fore finger with a scissor.*
>
> *There was no clinic nearby or hospital back then, so I got no help. Dada (owner of the house) gave his old handkerchief to stop the blood. Injection was given a day later. We have to keep ourselves in good health as it would be difficult for us to get any medical aid easily. I have heard they don't treat us nicely there so most times I self-medicate or ask a nearby pharmacist or ask other sisters what to take. I think if I would be living in the city in a more developed place I would not be speaking all this.* (Sumit, 44, Transgender man, Urban)

Those days were a lesson that real support must stop just short of alleviating purely psychological suffering and address the broader social and systemic inequities that maintain marginalization. In these moments of vulnerability and candid disclosure, she realized that effective research must strive to be transformative, actively working to dismantle oppressive systems while simultaneously validating and empowering marginalized voices.

This dual commitment, to scientific rigor and to social change, has since become the cornerstone of any research philosophy. The authors have embraced an advocacy-oriented research paradigm that is explicitly designed to inform public policy, enhance community awareness, and drive systemic reforms aimed at promoting inclusion and social justice. In doing so, the role of scholar-activist has crystallized for her. She now sees herself not just as an academic but as an active participant in the larger struggle for transgender rights and social justice, a struggle that calls for working across disciplines, honest and brave conversations, and a long-term commitment to truly understanding lived experiences in all their depth and complexity.

Rethinking Identity

In transgender research, as per the author's understanding, ontology is about recognizing that gender isn't fixed or limited to a binary, but exists as a spectrum of lived experiences. Epistemology then considers how we come to understand these experiences, through medical diagnoses, surveys, or, more importantly, the voices and stories of transgender people themselves. Knowledge production happens where these meet: when researchers design studies, write findings, or influence policy, they decide which realities are acknowledged and which ways of knowing are valued. For example, an approach that understands transgender identities mainly through "gender dysphoria" creates very different knowledge than community-based research that ponders upon resilience, culture, and lived experience. The journey she has undertaken has also led to important theoretical insights regarding identity formation and the meaning of belonging, particularly in a socio-cultural milieu as complex as India's.

For example, the theory of transgender congruence, a state of psychological flourishing based on matching between one's internal gender identity and external expression, has frequently been criticized as overly simplistic when applied to non-western settings (Pandya & Radcay, 2021). In India, where transgender identities are always embedded in a matrix of cultural tradition, collective rituals, and community hierarchy, such ideas fall short. Rather, the lived experiences of most transgender people uncover that psychological health is more entwined with social acceptance, economic security, and empowerment arising from collective identity formation.

> *We are rich or poor on a daily basis. When I have to work in the evening after 6:30 I have a good client. Sometimes I am rich, or suppose there is a child born nearby and they have given me handsome money. I am rich then, the next day I am poor. You think at your own end, if I were a boy or a girl in this country I know it would be challenging for girls but not nowadays, but won't it be easier for these genders to continue education?*
>
> *Won't it be easier to find a job, find a partner? To have a family, to be someone's son or daughter for life? Fighting on a daily basis for bread, clothes and house (roti kapda makaan in hindi) troubles us daily, the challenge was worsened in COVID though. Being a transgender in India is a task in itself, but I have listened to my mind always, I know I am out of the trap of either being a boy or girl but that being either of them would have brought stability in life, there would be less or no challenges if I haven't accepted my feeling and continued to being a boy.* (Kanti, 37, Transgender Woman, Urban)

> *I am coming from a lower background, so we never had enough resources. My father is a mason, and my mother is a housewife, with four sons, one daughter, and one me. So, it is hard coming from this background and having enough money for healthcare. I am glad that the government has policies to cover my health expenses up to a certain limit.* (Priya, 27, Transgender Woman, Urban)

Furthermore, the theoretical implications extend to the critique of medical and legal paradigms that have historically pathologized transgender identities. It has become increasingly clear that any meaningful theory of transgender identity in India must be grounded in an intersectional analysis, one that acknowledges the interplay of gender, caste, class, and regional identity while also remaining actively engaged with activist constituencies.

Community Engagement and the Path Forward

These interactions have traditionally been in the form of collaborative workshops, focus groups, and research projects in which trans persons take an active role in conceptualizing research questions, interpreting findings, and working on advocacy strategies. In these participatory processes, the dualism between research and lived experience has unfolded over time and has been replaced by a more integrated conceptualization, one that affirms the agency and competence of members of the community. This collaborative approach is a tool to the power of research founded on everyday realities, imbued with a commitment to equity, and committed to creating social justice. In addition to developing a better understanding of the research around Indian transgender persons, the author's' path has had profound implications for community empowerment and participation. At the core of this transformation has been the transition from researching transgender communities to openly collaborating with them. Participatory community-based research has allowed her to witness firsthand the hope, strength, and imagination that are fostered in the face of systematic oppression. She has seen directly how communities unite to create safe spaces, establish support systems, and speak in common voices about visions of social change. This co-creative process has not only enriched my scholarship but has reinforced the ethical imperative that scholarship can and must be a force for positive social transformation.

Reflections

Looking back on her journey from a bachelor's student of psychology to a researcher committed to advocacy, she has come to see how personal engagement and academic work can strengthen and enrich each other. What began as a quest to understand human behavior through standardized measures gradually transformed into an empathetic journey through the complex terrains of identity, culture, and resistance. This shift was not an easy one and it was accompanied by numerous challenges that the author had to confront her own prejudices, challenge established assumptions, and embrace the ambiguity that arises from participant-driven research. But it also allowed her to have the clarity of realizing that authentic social change occurs when solid scholarship combines with authentic community engagement. In this process, the author learned that research is never politically or socially neutral; it is imbued with values, ethical commitments, and the potential to change lives. By centering the experiences of transgender individuals in India, the author has come to understand that our lived realities, however painful, are also sites of resistance, innovation, and hope.

Implications for Future Research and Advocacy

Looking ahead one can see psychology, intersectionality, and advocacy coming together to open a new chapter in transgender studies. The journey has shown that scholarship must be more than theory; it must also create real social change. Future research needs to keep exploring the diverse and layered realities of transgender life while also addressing the urgent challenges of discrimination in terms of economic exclusion and limited healthcare faced by transgender communities in India. It is still vital to use participatory approaches. Researchers need to keep working closely with communities so their voices guide the questions, shape the findings, and influence policy. This way research not only adds to scholarship but also gives power back to those whose lives have long been silenced by dominant narratives. By consistent involvement, we can help develop customized interventions whether clinical, educational, or legal that value the cultural specificity, resilience, and dignity of transgender populations. Collaboration among various disciplines is called for in such an integrative approach. Psychologists, sociologists, legal scholars, and community organizers should collaborate to bring reprisal to the discourse surrounding transgender issues in India. With research based on qualitative data and community action along with policy analysis, reforms can be brought forth that would allow for better accessibility to quality healthcare, education, and opportunities of employment for transgender persons (Saraff et al., 2022). These partnerships might as well contest the enduring social stigmatization and legal hurdles that have furthered the marginalization of the communities, clearing the road toward equity.

How Do We Sum Up the Understanding of Transgender Realities?

The journey into transgender studies has been about shifts in the mindset and objectives. Having come from the well-defined but narrow confines of conventional social psychology, the author has embraced a very expanded, intersectional approach to research, which is advocacy-oriented. This journey has taught her that the statistical abstractions of the generalized method she adhered to aren't the only ones she should use to represent the vibrancy, anguish, and resilience experienced by individuals who are transgender in India. Once she understands their plea then she can go ahead with a larger set of data and use relevant statistics. Deep engagement with these stories nourishes her academic undertaking while forcing her to rethink the role of the scholar as someone empathetic and active in the struggle for social justice. In retrospect, each step of academic evolution, from the earlier days of reliance on quantitative models to later days of embracing community-based participatory methods, has been informed by increasing acknowledgment of the power that is inherent in lived experience. Indeed, participation of transgender people via interviews, forums, or daily life encounters has broadened this discussion relating to identity, exclusion, and resilience. These encounters reminded her that the research process should not just be about theories or knowledge production; it must equally be about catalyzing change and empowering people as a way of opposing oppressive structures. As she looks ahead, she is still committed to promoting transgender studies along both scientifically rigorous and humanistic lines. While penning this chapter, the author felt that she is sharing a personal reflection and a call to action. She hopes this chapter creates the need to rethink research methods so they truly honor the complexities of gender, identity, and social diversity. In doing so, it adds to the wider push, both in academia and society, for greater inclusivity, cultural sensitivity, and rights-based advocacy. The hope is very simple—the insights from this journey not only inspire future researchers like you, but also spark real social change that uplifts transgender communities and transforms their everyday lives.

References

Arvind, A., Pandya, A., Amin, L., Aggarwal, M., Agrawal, D., Tiwari, K., et al. (2022). Social strain, distress, and gender dysphoria among transgender women and Hijra in Vadodara. *India. International Journal of Transgender Health, 23*(1–2), 149–163.

Ata, N., Chaudhary, S., & Kulshrestha, T. (2025). A policy discourse analysis of educational provisions for the transgender community in India. *Educational Review*, 1–21.

Balabantaray, S. R., & Singh, A. (2022). Review of (revisiting) the transgender education in India: An analysis of the National Educational Policy 2020. *Journal of Public Affairs, 22*(2), e2504.

Baudh, S. (2013). Decriminalisation of consensual same-sex sexual acts in the South Asian Commonwealth: Struggles in contexts. In *Human rights, sexual orientation and gender identity in the Commonwealth* (pp. 287–312). University of London Press.

Ben-Ari, A., & Enosh, G. (2011). Processes of reflectivity: Knowledge construction in qualitative research. *Qualitative Social Work, 10*(2), 152–171.

Bhaskaran, S. (2013). The politics of penetration: Section 377 of the Indian Penal Code. In *Queering India* (pp. 15–29). Routledge.

Bhattacharya, S., & Ghosh, D. (2020). Studying physical and mental health status among hijra, kothi and transgender community in Kolkata, India. *Social Science & Medicine, 265*, 113412.

Bhattacharya, S., Ghosh, D., & Purkayastha, B. (2022). 'Transgender persons (protection of rights) act' of India: An analysis of substantive access to rights of a transgender community. *Journal of Human Rights Practice, 14*(2), 676–697.

Boskey, E. R. (2014). Understanding transgender identity development in childhood and adolescence. *American Journal of Sexuality Education, 9*(4), 445–463.

Chandra, S. (2017). Transgender Children's education and their reengagement in society. *International Journal of Educational Research Studies, 2*(13), 875–890.

Clark, C. T., Lo, R. S., & Chen, J. (2025). Queerness. In *Children's literature and culture* (pp. 55–69). Routledge.

Collins, S. E., Clifasefi, S. L., Stanton, J., The Leap Advisory Board, Straits, K. J. E., Gil-Kashiwabara, E., Rodriguez Espinosa, P., Nicasio, A. V., Andrasik, M. P., Hawes, S. M., Miller, K. A., Nelson, L. A., Orfaly, V. E., Duran, B. M., & Wallerstein, N. (2018, October). Community-based participatory research (CBPR): Towards equitable involvement of community in psychology research. *American Psychologist, 73*(7), 884–898. https://doi.org/10.1037/amp0000167

Crenshaw, K. (1991). Mapping the margins: Intersectionality, identity politics, and violence against Women of color, 43 stanford law review 1241-99. In *Women of color at the center: Selections from the Third National Conference on Women of Color and the Law.*

Das, R. (2025). *Messy Trans and Queer Storytelling: (Un) Doing Indian Exceptionalism* (Doctoral dissertation, The University of Iowa).

Gupta, A. (2006). Section 377 and the dignity of Indian homosexuals. *Economic and Political Weekly*, 4815–4823.

Hauge, Å. L. (2007). Identity and place: A critical comparison of three identity theories. *Architectural Science Review, 50*(1), 44–51.

Hossain, A. (2017). Section 377, same-sex sexualities and the struggle for sexual rights in Bangladesh. *Australian Journal of Asian Law, 20*, 115.

Jain, D. (2022). Right to health and gender-affirmative procedure in the Transgender Persons Act 2019 in India. *Indian Journal of Plastic Surgery, 55*(02), 205–210.

Jain, D., Aggarwal, N., Ray, K., Karwa, S., Chaudhari, D., & Devrani, R. (2025). Education equity for transgender and gender-diverse persons in India: Insights into implementation Hurdles. *Michigan Journal of Gender & Law, 32*(1), 1–100.

Kalra, G. (2012). Hijras: The unique transgender culture of India. *International Journal of Culture and Mental Health, 5*(2), 121–126.

Kaur, H., & Singh, T. A. (2024). Qualitative Exploration of the role of intersectionality in health disparities faced by Indian transgender persons. *Psychology Hub, 41*, 23–34. https://doi.org/10.13133/2724-2943/18227

Mazumdar, M. (2016). *Hijra Lives: Negotiating social exclusion and identities.* Tata Institute of Social Sciences.

Mehta, R. (2021). Analysing transgender rights in India. *Indian Journal of Law and Legal Research, 2*, 1.

Mukherjee, A. (2023). *Exploring the social and political lives of gender nonconforming people in India* (Doctoral dissertation, Newcastle University).

Nizza, I. E., Farr, J., & Smith, J. A. (2021). Achieving excellence in interpretative phenomenological analysis (IPA): Four markers of high quality. *Qualitative Research in Psychology, 18*(3), 369–386.

Opia, F. N., & Matthew, K. A. (2025). Empowering unrepresented populations through inclusive policy frameworks in global health initiatives. *International Journal of Modern Science and Research Technology, 7*(1). https://doi.org/10.56726/IRJMETS66444

Page, K. (2022). Ethics and the co-production of knowledge. *Public Health Research and Practice, 32*(2). https://doi.org/10.17061/phrp3222213

Page, S., Burgess, J., Davies-Abbott, I., Roberts, D., & Molderson, J. (2016). Transgender, mental health, and older people: An appreciative approach towards working together. *Issues in Mental Health Nursing, 37*(12), 903–911.

Pandya, A. K., & Redcay, A. (2021). Access to health services: Barriers faced by the transgender population in India. *Journal of Gay & Lesbian Mental Health, 25*(2), 132–154.

Pinna, F., Paribello, P., Somaini, G., Corona, A., Ventriglio, A., Corrias, C., et al. (2022). Mental health in transgender individuals: A systematic review. *International Review of Psychiatry, 34*(3–4), 292–359.

Saraff, S., Singh, T., Kaur, H., & Biswal, R. (2022). Stigma and health of Indian LGBT population: A systematic review. *Stigma Health, 7*, 178–195.

Singh, T., Kaur, H., & Mittal, S. (2023). Sexual orientation and gender identity and school life in India. In *SOGI minority and school life in Asian contexts* (pp. 156–170). Routledge.

Singh, T., Tushir, B., Mittal, S., & Kaur, H. (2024). Unveiling health disparities: Navigating the unique challenges faced by abused women, transgender individuals, and underprivileged children. In P. Liamputtong (Ed.), *Handbook of concepts in health, health behavior and environmental health*. Springer. https://doi.org/10.1007/978-981-97-0821-5_145-1

Smith, J. A. (2011). Evaluating the contribution of interpretative phenomenological analysis. *Health Psychology Review, 5*(1), 9–27.

Smith, J. A. (2017). Interpretative phenomenological analysis: Getting at lived experience. *The Journal of Positive Psychology, 12*(3), 303–304.

Soohinda, G., Jaggi, P. S., Sampath, H., Bhardwaj, A., & Dutta, S. (2025). Freedom and healing: Did the decriminalization of homosexuality impact the mental health of gay men in India? An Online Survey. *Journal of Homosexuality, 13*, 1–16.

Srivastava, A., & Kumar, V. (2019). Section 377 and LGBT activism in India. *International Journal of Research and Analytical Reviews, 6*(2), 30–34.
Waggy, M. M., & Bashir, D. (2025). Transgender rights in India's legal system: A critical analysis. *Sexuality Research and Social Policy, 22*(1), 101–107.
Wallerstein, N. B., & Duran, B. (2006). Using community-based participatory research to address health disparities. *Health promotion practice, 7*(3), 312–323. https://doi.org/10.1177/1524839906289376

3

Ethical Considerations and Collaborative Research

Abstract Framed within critical research ethics, this chapter examines the imperative of conducting respectful and equitable research with transgender communities in India. It critiques extractive research models and advocates for a paradigm shift from researcher-as-observer to researcher-as-collaborator. The discussion focuses on practical strategies for safeguarding participant dignity through informed consent, confidentiality, and the mindful navigation of power dynamics. It outlines methods for building sustained trust, practicing cultural humility, and ensuring community ownership of the research process and its outcomes. The chapter serves as a guide for ethical engagement, positing that the highest value of research lies in its capacity to empower communities and contribute to positive social transformation.

Keywords Research ethics • Informed consent • Power dynamics • Collaborative research • Cultural humility • Data confidentiality • Empowerment • Ethical frameworks

H. Kaur, *Psychological Research Among Transgender Individuals*,
https://doi.org/10.1007/978-3-032-12051-9_3

Transgender communities in India are made up of people with diverse identities, experiences and histories and studying them calls for research that is deeply ethical, collaborative and culturally grounded (Chakrapani, 2010; Chakrapani et al., 2007, 2018, 2023). In this chapter, we explore the ethical imperatives and collaborative strategies for conducting research with transgender communities, drawing on established frameworks, such as the Helsinki Guidelines, Belmont Report and the CIOMS guidelines, that prioritize respect for persons, beneficence, and justice. This discussion is rooted in the Indian context where stigma marginalization and unequal power deeply shape both lived experiences and the way research is done. We will explore these questions in the following parts: *Safeguarding dignity from observer to collaborator, building bridges of trust* and *an open invitation to co-create the future of transgender research.*

Safeguarding Dignity: The Imperative of Ethical Research?

As discussed before, marginalized groups especially transgender communities in India live at the crossroads of stigma, legal barriers, and systemic discrimination which makes them particularly vulnerable in research settings (Saraff et al., 2022). Researchers have an ethical duty to recognize this from the start and design their work in ways that protect the dignity and rights of participants (Arvind et al., 2021). Respect for persons means seeing transgender individuals not as subjects of study but as human beings with rights whose autonomy must always be honored. Next is getting informed consent, which is a core part of doing ethical research and with transgender communities it is especially important that the process is transparent and sensitive to context (Elischberger et al., 2018). A true informed consent means explaining the purpose of the study in simple, clear language without jargon and making sure it is fully understandable for people with different levels of formal education. Researchers must commit to a dynamic consent process wherein participants are provided opportunities to ask questions, express concerns, and withdraw consent at any stage without fear of retribution. In doing so, the researcher fosters an environment in which participants feel empowered and respected as autonomous individuals. Because transgender identities and healthcare information are so sensitive it is crucial to protect privacy and confidentiality at every stage of the research (Chandra, 2017; Shaikh et al., 2016). This means using secure ways to store data removing all personal identifiers and limiting access to sensitive information while also being open with participants about how their data will be used. Even a small accidental disclosure of someone's transgender status can cause serious social or legal harm which makes confidentiality a non-negotiable part of ethical research. This responsibility becomes even greater in places with weak legal protections and high levels of stigma where researchers must use both technological and practical safeguards to keep participants safe.

In this ethical compliance, it is vital to address the power imbalance between researchers and transgender participants if we want to build a research space that is truly respectful and collaborative. Traditional research often puts the researcher in control but ethical research calls for sharing that power and involving participants in decisions. Using community advisory boards and participatory methods can make this possible while reminding researchers to stay aware of their own privilege. This balance also requires constant self-reflection so that the process values the lived experiences and knowledge of transgender communities as much as academic expertise.

From Observer to Collaborator: Redefining Researcher Roles

The shift from being a distant observer to becoming a true partner in research is a transformative one and it takes deep personal reflection and a strong commitment to ethics. Early in her career, the author saw the limits of extractive research that focused only on collecting data without giving back to the community. She witnessed the mistrust that such practices created. Moving toward a collaborative approach meant working with transgender community leaders, taking part in community events, and letting their voices shape the research itself. This change is not just a professional responsibility; it is also a moral duty when working with marginalized communities. Community-driven research means giving ownership of the process back to transgender communities and working with them to shape the questions, design the methods and make sense of the findings. Approaches like CBPR are powerful because they are built on reciprocity and equal collaboration. When community members are treated not just as participants but as co researchers the work becomes more meaningful. The questions reflect real needs and the methods respect local culture. This way research creates a sense of empowerment and ownership and the outcomes are not only more accurate but also more likely to lead to real change.

Bringing community knowledge and lived experience into research design is one of the strongest ways to make sure the work is ethical and meaningful. Transgender participants carry insights from their own lives that are often missing in traditional research. When researchers include these stories in their work they not only challenge dominant narratives but also help build these perspectives essential for creating interventions that are culturally sensitive and truly effective (Chakrapani et al., 2017; Pandya & Redcay, 2021). For example, qualitative studies show that community advocacy and culturally rooted practices like cultural clapping play a key role in how transgender people negotiate access to healthcare (Kaur & Singh, 2024; Parmenter et al., 2021). When researchers include these stories in their work they not only challenge dominant narratives but also help build evidence that is richer, more nuanced, and validated by the community itself.

A key part of moving from observer to collaborator is being willing to face and unlearn our own biases. Researchers have to look closely at how their assumptions about gender sexuality and identity shape the way they see data and engage with participants. This takes honest self- reflection and ongoing dialogue with transgender community members whose lived experiences offer valuable corrections. Approaching research with humility and openness makes the work stronger both ethically and scientifically while also challenging the hierarchies that have long silenced transgender voices.

Building Bridges of Trust—Cultivating Strong Relationships

Real collaboration begins with active listening and open non-judgmental communication. These are the foundations of trust with transgender communities. Researchers must create spaces both physical and virtual, where people feel truly safe to share their stories without fear. Listening deeply is more than hearing words, it is about understanding the cultural and emotional layers that give them meaning. Open communication being honest about the purpose, risks, and outcomes of the research helps make the process clear and builds lasting trust. India is a diverse fabric; we speak very different languages and uphold very different religions and cultures and yet remain united. This is our identity and we take pride in it; therefore, as researchers we should be sensitive and humble. Cultural sensitivity means truly understanding the diverse traditions, beliefs, and practices within transgender communities in India. Researchers need to go beyond showing respect and actively weave these cultural nuances into the design of their studies so that methods and interventions fit the local context. Humility is key here; it means recognizing the limits of our own perspective and turning to community experts for guidance. In practice this could look like co-creating research tools with transgender leaders or adapting consent forms to more local languages and to different literacy levels.

Typically, the scientist should be able to account for transparency when dealing with a vulnerable section of society in research. Transparency should shine at all levels: in decisions related to funding, choice of methods, presentation of outcome results, and final report of the study. Feedback loops must also be established so that community members get an opportunity to review and respond to the findings before being further shared. Accountability also means that data must be protected with care through stringent security measures and confidentiality and that participants should be fully informed on how their data will be kept from harm. At the core of ethical research lies the principle that the benefits must directly reach the communities involved (American Psychological Association, 2015). Community ownership is realized, for instance, when transgender persons are included as co-investigators on research projects, advisory board members, and even in disseminating the findings of research. This presence fortifies the validity of the research among the culturally relevant population while simultaneously fostering community empowerment through capacity-building with shared goals. Training workshops and skill-building sessions in educational outreach are good examples where trained participants act as social change agents contributing simultaneously to the knowledge base. These models, thus, tether research outcomes with actual benefits such as improving access to healthcare or initiation of advocacy for policy changes that purposely address and lessen the structural inequities meted out to transgender communities.

Co-creating the Future of Transgender Research

The traditional notion of data extraction must lose its charm and give way to the imperative for joint creations and collaborations. Researchers are required not only to collect data but to engage in the reflective process that examines whose knowledge counts, who benefits from the research, and how the research is concretely applied in the real world. The ethical imperative in these scenarios is that research shall empower rather than exploit transgender communities; therefore, this should be viewed as an attempt to shift from extractive toward mutually beneficial engagements (Vincent, 2018). Furtherance of research that is scientifically innovative and morally mature is critical in embracing such collaborative approaches as CBPR. These participatory methods engage transgender community members along the entire research continuum from conceptualization, design, implementation through to dissemination so that the research evolves around the community needs and in response to their lived experiences (American Psychological Association, 2015). Community-based data collection methods, including respondent-driven sampling and focus group discussions within safe community spaces, have proven effective in recruiting hard-to-reach populations while simultaneously building trust and mitigating power imbalances.

One foremost ethical concern in research with transgender populations is ensuring that the welfare of the community is placed above any form of academic or individual ambition. The researchers must have a critical mindset and determine if their work either sustains or even undermines the dignity, rights, and well-being of the trans communities, rather than serving as simply providing scholarly knowledge. This change in ideology really emphasizes rejecting hierarchical research models that put academic output at the center and endorsing long-term community benefits such as better healthcare services, policy advocacy, or empowerment by educational means. Researchers can operationalize this commitment by ensuring that every stage of the research process, from fieldwork through data analysis and dissemination, involves mechanisms for reciprocal benefit and that community feedback is incorporated as an ongoing corrective measure (American Psychological Association, 2015).

With an eye to the future, a prospective research avenue is seen where transgender communities are front and center in defining their developmental trajectories and the interventions best suited to their help. The vision requires an amalgamation of collaborative, community-led approaches that value transparency, accountability, and mutual respect. Transformation in research goes further than just questions and methodologies to ensure that transgender communities themselves interpret and disseminate findings so that the narratives are "by and for" with and by the community. Co-owning their research outputs gives transgender communities the leverage to use scientific knowledge as a basis for advocacy and policy changes around the structural inequities that have long entrenched their marginalization (Kohout-Diaz, 2025; Vincent, 2018).

The ethical conduct of research among transgender communities requires, among several other parameters, respect for persons, beneficence, and justice as embodied in the international ethical frameworks such as the Belmont Report and the CIOMS guidelines (CIOMS). This chapter has elaborated strategies to protect dignity through informed consent processes, strong confidentiality provisions, and engagement that continuously assesses and addresses power imbalances. Moving from merely watching to collaborating places interest in research of the community and co-created knowledge that voice real-life experiences in social justice. They have created bridges of trust through open communication, cultural sensitivity, and joint ownership in the research process that empowers not only the research but the transgender communities.

In light of this, researchers are called upon to take their methodology toward co-creation over extractive practices with community well-being at its core. This means to inherently uphold participatory ways as a matter of worldview and ethical responsibility while critically interrogating one's own assumptions. Only then will the work become truly transformative, just, and inclusive in working with transgender communities.

As we move forward the call is clear: we must break down the power imbalances built into traditional research, support community-led agendas, and commit to research that is transparent, accountable, and culturally sensitive (Vincent, 2018). Research should not just produce knowledge but bring real and lasting benefits for transgender communities in India and beyond. In doing so, we contribute not only to the academic literature but to the broader struggle for justice, equity, and recognition of transgender identities as it exists in the real world. In closing the vision is simple but powerful, an inclusive research space built on respect, trust, and shared knowledge (Kohout-Diaz, 2025). Such a space will not only move science forward but also help build a more just and equal society where transgender communities shape the research questions, guide the methods, and share ownership of their own stories. This is the future we must create together—a future where ethical research becomes a bridge connecting academic rigor with community empowerment making sure that every step in knowledge directly supports the well-being and self-determination of transgender communities in India and beyond.

References

American Psychological Association. (2015). Guidelines for psychological practice with transgender and gender nonconforming people. *American Psychologist, 70*(9), 832–864.

Arvind, A., Pandya, A., Amin, L., Aggarwal, M., Agrawal, D., Tiwari, K., Singh, S., Nemkul, M., & Agarwal, P. (2021). Social strain, distress, and gender dysphoria among transgender women and Hijra in Vadodara, India. *International Journal of Transgender Health, 23*(1-2), 149–163. https://doi.org/10.1080/26895269.2020.1845273

Belmont Report. (n.d.). https://www.hhs.gov/ohrp/regulations-and-policy/belmont-report/read-the-bel mont-report/index.html

Chakrapani, V. (2010). *Hijras/transgender women in India: HIV, human rights and social exclusion.* United Nations Development Programme.

Chakrapani, V., Newman, P. A., & Noronha, E. (2018). Hijras/transwomen and sex work in India. In *Transgender sex work and society* (pp. 214–235). Harrington Park Press.

Chakrapani, V., Newman, P. A., Shunmugam, M., McLuckie, A., & Melwin, F. (2007). Structural violence against kothi–identified men who have sex with men in Chennai, India: A qualitative investigation. *AIDS Education & Prevention, 19*(4), 346–364.

Chakrapani, V., Newman, P. A., Shunmugam, M., Rawat, S., Mohan, B. R., Baruah, D., & Tepjan, S. (2023). A scoping review of lesbian, gay, bisexual, transgender, queer, and intersex (LGBTQI+) people's health in India. *PLOS Global Public Health, 3*(4), e0001362.

Chakrapani, V., Vijin, P. P., Logie, C. H., Newman, P. A., Shunmugam, M., Sivasubramanian, M., & Samuel, M. (2017). Understanding how sexual and gender minority stigmas influence depression among trans women and men who have sex with men in India. *LGBT Health, 4*(3), 217–226.

Chandra, S. (2017). Transgender Children's education and their reengagement in society. *International Journal of Educational Research Studies, 2*(13), 875–890.

CIOMS. (n.d.). https://cioms.ch/wp-content/uploads/2017/01/WEB-CIOMS-EthicalGuidelines.pdf

Elischberger, H. B., Glazier, J. J., Hill, E. D., & Verduzco-Baker, L. (2018). Attitudes toward and beliefs about transgender youth: A cross-cultural comparison between the United States and India. *Sex roles, 78*(1), 142–160.

Helsinki Guidelines. (n.d.). https://www.wma.net/policies-post/wma-declaration-of-helsinki/

Kaur, H., & Singh, T. A. (2024). Qualitative Exploration of the role of intersectionality in health disparities faced by Indian transgender persons. *Psychology Hub, 41*, 23–34. https://doi.org/10.13133/2724-2943/18227

Kohout-Diaz, M. (2025). Advancing an inclusive research approach in humanities and social sciences: The crucial role of self-study and narrative enquiry in doctoral research experiences. *Social Sciences & Humanities Open, 11*, 101256.

Pandya, A. K., & Redcay, A. (2021). Access to health services: Barriers faced by the transgender population in India. *Journal of Gay & Lesbian Mental Health, 25*(2), 132–154.

Parmenter, J. G., Galliher, R. V., Wong, E., & Perez, D. (2021). An intersectional approach to understanding LGBTQ+ people of color's access to LGBTQ+ community resilience. *Journal of Counseling Psychology, 68*(6), 629.

Saraff, S., Singh, T., Kaur, H., & Biswal, R. (2022). Stigma and health of Indian LGBT population: A systematic review. *Stigma Health, 7*, 178–195.

Shaikh, S., Mburu, G., Arumugam, V., Mattipalli, N., Aher, A., Mehta, S., & Robertson, J. (2016). Empowering communities and strengthening systems to improve transgender health: Outcomes from the Pehchan programme in India. *Journal of the International AIDS Society, 19*, 20809.

Vincent, B. W. (2018). Studying trans: Recommendations for ethical recruitment and collaboration with transgender participants in academic research. *Psychology & Sexuality, 9*(2), 102–116.

4

Designing and Conducting Inclusive Research

Abstract This chapter details the methodological framework for designing and implementing inclusive research practices. It argues for the adaptation of traditional data collection methods, such as interviews, surveys, and observation that is to be more accessible, comfortable, and culturally competent for diverse participants, with a specific focus on transgender communities. The author shares concrete techniques for creating safe interview environments, employing sensitive language, and practicing active listening. The chapter also addresses the analytical phase, emphasizing the role of critical reflexivity in interpreting data and the importance of narrative storytelling to honor the depth of lived experience. The central idea is that inclusivity is not merely a procedural step but a fundamental philosophy that should infuse every stage of the research process.

Keywords Inclusive methodology • Qualitative research • Interview techniques • Cultural competence • Active listening • Reflexivity • Data analysis • Narrative storytelling • Participatory design

H. Kaur, *Psychological Research Among Transgender Individuals*,
https://doi.org/10.1007/978-3-032-12051-9_4

Here is a comprehensive understanding for designing and conducting inclusive research, specifically when encompassing transgender individuals. This chapter is organized into five major sections: an introduction to inclusive research, building inclusive research approaches (addressing diversity and effective data gathering methods), analyzing and interpreting data, storytelling and meaning-making, and a conclusion with a call to action. Each section combines what the author has seen in her research with frameworks already recognized in the literature as discussed in previous chapters.

Inclusive Research

Inclusive research is a multidimensional, participatory approach that challenges traditional researcher–subject hierarchies by actively involving community members in every phase of the research cycle (Singh et al., 2013). The idea is that communities hold valuable lived knowledge, and research strengthens when it respectfully includes voices across cultures, genders, socioeconomic backgrounds, and religions. The author's' work in social science research has spanned health, education, and community development projects (Forber-Pratt, 2024). The author has seen firsthand the benefits of unfolding research processes that respect participants as co-researchers instead of passive subjects. Research that is attentive to human differences expands the relevance of its findings by including diverse viewpoints. It also strengthens social justice and empowers communities by encouraging critical self-awareness and cultural humility (Forber-Pratt, 2024).

Inclusive research methods merge participatory approaches and reflexive evaluation to ethically and effectively respond to communities' requirements, tastes, and cultural frameworks. Based on the observations, inclusivity is dynamic and depends on commitment, community appreciation, and self-evaluation during the design, data collection, and analysis stages (Divan et al., 2016). This can be seen as insights to be used for designing and conducting research which aims to foster inclusivity. One can find the text below useful how to adapt the approach to thoughtfully engage differences in gender, religion, socioeconomic background, and other social identities. The aim is to ensure that every person's perspective is collected, honored, and amplified.

Building Inclusive Research Approaches

A researcher committed to inclusive work understands that one can't just study people without seeing them in their full complexity. They know that a person's background, their gender, their faith, their financial situation, their racial identity, or whether they are transgender or have a disability, fundamentally shapes how they move through the world and, in turn, how they might experience a research study. Taking a project on health disparities, for example, a researcher might notice that the usual method to select participants picks out only one particular segment. That researcher then actively looks for new methods. Using local community leaders or advertising in places favored by underrepresented groups is a great way to widen the reach. This approach is not to tick off on a checklist but to engage with the community, which is rarely heard. All researchers have a pile of data to collect. Still, in this case, a conscious effort is made to collect data mixed with meaningful context and stories so that the picture the researcher is trying to paint is complete. The solution is relatable to the community (Rosenberg & Tilley, 2021).

To gain insight into somebody, we need to analyze the unique composition of their identity, such as their occupation, gender, religion, race, and the way all of these intersect to influence a person's life. Intersectional perspective is adoptive to understand the subject thoroughly in such research. It requires me to consider how many identities construct a person's life instead of reducing them to a singular one. For example, instead of employing a standard questionnaire which can only permit "male" and "female" responses, permit transgender, non-binary, and genderqueer. This seems like a trivial adjustment, but it's meaningful. The information thus reflects actual lives, rather than omitting or distorting individuals (Divan et al., 2016; Elischberger et al., 2018; Thomas et al., 2017).

Changing research methods to cater to a community's mixed nature means constantly thinking of creating an inclusive culture for all members. While working with people of varying social and economic ranks, one has had to change interview frameworks and methods of taking consent multiple times. Working with community leaders has helped. Use simple language that does not contain unnecessary university-level words, as is common in the use of language among people employed in educational and research institutions. Such an adjustment is not cosmetic but maintains the essential respect that participants deserve and encourages them to tell their stories without judging or misrepresenting them.

Gathering Information

The methodological basis of inclusive research is rooted in carefully selecting and adjusting data collection methods. Structured interviews, focus groups, surveys, and participant observation are all routinely utilized methods that can be adjusted to accommodate the heterogeneous needs of research participants. While working on research projects, the author used qualitative and quantitative data collection methods, emphasizing accessibility. For instance, when the participants of your research are coming from geographical divisions or are hailing from different socioeconomic backgrounds, or are time bound and couldn't afford time for meeting, one should conduct interviews through telephone. Similarly, if others face technological barriers and are not open to talk over telephone and don't wish to get recorded one can go for face-to-face interviews (Miles & Huberman, 1994).

Furthermore, by providing explicit, jargon-free materials, one can ensure that survey instruments are understandable to people of different educational backgrounds, which enhances both response rates and data quality. A key component of data gathering is the implementation of culturally competent interview techniques, particularly when engaging with transgender individuals. Establishing a safe, respectful environment in which participants feel heard, respected, and seen is key. Drawing on experience and informed by the literature, the following practical strategies are effective for the author when interviewing transgender participants.

Use Preferred Language and Pronouns

Before beginning the interview, ascertain and use each participant's name and pronoun. This establishes respect from the outset and communicates that the researcher is committed to meeting participants on their own terms. Create a comfortable interview environment. Whether the interview is in-person or virtual, select locations and setups that ensure privacy and comfort. In my research, I have arranged interviews in venues that are accessible, informal, and free from distractions, which has significantly eased participants' anxieties (Braybrook et al., 2023).

Offer Flexibility in Communication Modes

Recognizing that some transgender individuals may prefer written responses or asynchronous communication due to past experiences with discrimination, one should alternate between face-to-face interviews, video calls, and secure written exchanges, thereby removing pressure and allowing participants to communicate in the way that serves them best. Training in cultural competence is indispensable. In every interview, one should explicitly reference the importance of participants' lived experiences and validate their narratives with empathetic questioning and reflective listening. This practice builds rapport and encourages deeper, more honest exchanges. Moreover, collaboration with recognized community stakeholders, such as working with transgender advocacy organizations, increases credibility and assists in recruitment and continued involvement. This collaborative approach honors the belief that individuals who belong to the community are experts on their own lives and promotes genuinely inclusive research collaborations. One should practice this as it enhances the ethical integrity and helps in maintaining a sound standard of methodology.

Analyzing and Interpreting Data

The inclusivity commitment also proceeds into the analysis stage, where researchers need to reflect on their biases and positionality factors that may affect the interpretation of data. A cycle of reflexivity, iterative checking, and consultation with communities has been central to my data analysis strategy in inclusive research.

Opinion on Arguments

Beginning with a one- or two-sentence defensive and specific claim statement, which is both considerable and precise, is the first step toward transforming an opinion on transgender research into an academic argument. Personal belief should be substituted with the most relevant empirical evidence, such as mental health, and sociological, psychological, or other subject-specific peer-reviewed studies, to verify and support the claim rigorously. Starting with a single- or two-sentence specific and defensive claim statement, both significant and accurate, is the first move to turn an opinion on transgender studies into an academic argument. Personal conviction has to be replaced with the most acceptable and pertinent empirical evidence, such as gender dysphoria, mental health, or sociological peer-reviewed studies, to confirm and authenticate the claim strictly. The argument should be constructed using analytical writing, where the argument is explained coherently, counterarguments are considered and evaluated, which adds to the credibility of the position, and the fairness is exhibited in the gracious tone of concession. Finally, the language must be precise. Evidence should be permitted appropriately tentatively, and emotive or biased phrasing should be avoided, so the conclusion is offered as a reasoned prescription rather than an opinion (Cottrell, 2023).

Having a Critical Reflection

We are often taught to develop critical thinking skills and be academic writers. The question is, how does one do crucial thinking for transgender research? Here I have penned two examples:

One of the poor critical reflections on transgender studies would start by somatically asserting, "I've always believed that being transgender is just a phase," and after interviewing one individual who detransitioned, "I know I'm right." This approach is founded upon one anecdote and individual opinion as its sole evidence, sidestepping all need to look at accepted medical consensus or the experienced existence of the vast majority of transgender people. The reflection would meander without direction, leaping from individual opinion to a cursory reference to a YouTube video without following it to its depth. It would avoid challenging terrain, such as the complex interplay of biology, identity, and social acceptance, and would completely ignore relevant theories from endocrinology, psychology, and sociology. The conclusion would be a foregone repetition of the initial prejudice, offering no new insight, demonstrating no criticality, and showing no ethical consideration for the confidentiality or dignity of the individuals used as examples. It remains a superficial description of a pre-held belief, unchanged by evidence or analysis. In the following paragraph one can understand a more thoughtful reflection (Cottrell, 2023).

First, the reflection would state clearly the main intention, for instance "this unravels my original concerns regarding gender-affirming care for teens, rooted in one case I came across, and contrasts it with the robust guidance provided by the new WPATH standards of care." It would take a responsible approach to tracing back the origin of the skepticism, perhaps there was an imbalance in the information, or a pattern of reportage within mass media to contrast with the very easy scapegoating of "those activists." It would take the complexity of the issue and assess in detail the clinical evidence on the two opposing sides: long-term studies of mental health outcomes and the debatable application of puberty blockers (Streed et al., 2023). Theory would be brought in appropriately, perhaps in an attempt to apply minority stress to explain increased anxiety in order to deconstruct the preconceived notions of the author. The work would cover rough ground and transparently wrestle with complicated ethical issues of autonomy and long-term impacts. The ending would not be a neat resolution but an array of carefully reasoned inferences: an enhanced appreciation of the necessity for personalized, evidence-based treatments, a promise to attend to the narratives of transgender people, and an acknowledgment and a recognition of the need for more research in specific areas. This demonstrates clear integrity, criticality, and a forward movement in understanding (Cottrell, 2023).

Dealing with Data Obtained

Reflexive thematic analysis is then utilized in the first instance to determine recurring patterns within the data, being sensitive to the contextual influences driving each participant's voice. Multiple coding rounds and the incorporation of deductive and inductive codes ensure themes arise organically from the data instead of being imposed too early. There is frequent reflective journaling to capture early interpretation and later re-examine these views in light of emerging participant insight.

Second, one can establish joint data review sessions with co-researchers and community advisers representing the various study groups. The sessions are not a formality but permit negotiation of meaning and avoid ascribing meanings by researchers based on their cultural background. For instance, in reviewing interviews with transgender participants, input from community members has been instrumental in sharpening categories and making sure that their everyday experiences are accurately represented. In the third place, it is essential to use methodological triangulation by integrating qualitative information with quantitative patterns (Moolchaem et al, 2015).

This study approach lets me validate the outcomes from different perspectives. The author gained a clear and unbiased understanding, which respects diversity, by ensuring a complete study by comparing and contrasting the survey, interview, and observational data results. In addition, do not forget that every analytical choice comes with a set of ethical concerns. For instance, ongoing scrutiny is applied to avoid misrepresenting words from the underrepresented communities with choices like data segmentation, variable aggregation, and narrative synthesis. As an example, one can explore the meaning of gender identities and socioeconomic factors, intentionally dealing with and trying to eliminate reductionist methods that hide the complex interactions of such matters. In summary, here the data analysis practices are underpinned by three major principles: reflexivity, triangulation, and collaborative interpretation. These strategies have consistently ensured that the conclusions drawn are inclusive, accurately represent the diversity of participant experiences, and are free from unwarranted researcher bias.

Understanding How Phenomenology Works for Transgender Persons

One analysis that the author thinks is a best fit for working with transgender persons and understanding their lived experience is IPA as discussed briefly in Chap. 2. It is a qualitative method to elucidate how participants interpret their lived experience. When engaging with transgender participants. It offers a method for collecting the richness and intricacy of individual accounts of gender identity, transition, relationships, and belonging. Researchers employing IPA are involved in a double hermeneutic process in which participants interpret their own experience, and researchers then interpret those interpreted meanings. This creates rich information about how transgender people experience themselves within cultural, medical, and interpersonal realities. By emphasizing rich, firsthand descriptions, IPA speaks to marginalized experience and illuminates the distinctive and heterogeneous way transgender individuals negotiate identity and meaning (Nizza et al., 2021; Smith, 2011, 2017).

Storytelling and Meaning-Making

Other than IPA, one can go into narrative inquiry. Compelling storytelling in inclusive research goes beyond merely presenting findings; it is a meaning-making process that respects and amplifies participants' voices. Throughout the authors' research insights, she has sought to create narrative spaces that honor participants' personal stories, enabling them to articulate their experiences in their own words. One approach that the author has successfully employed is participatory narrative inquiry. Participants can be invited to share their stories through open-ended interviews and written narratives, and the researcher can use methods such as story completion tasks to prompt the reflective accounts. It is certain that this approach empowers our participants to articulate their unique experiences and transforms data into co-constructed narratives that capture the complexities of identity and the given context (Nizza, Farr & Smith, 2021; Smith, 2011, 2017).

A crucial aspect of inclusive research is the utilization of appropriate dissemination methods. Even though they are valuable, traditional academic publications may fail to represent the full depth of lived experiences. To address this limitation if faced by the researcher, one can develop digital story maps, short digital documentaries, and interactive digital exhibitions, enabling people to experience the research findings more effectively, the enhanced versions of the symposium, conferences we hold now. Such dissemination methods ensure that the research is accessible to and culturally meaningful for non-academic publics, responding to the demands of inclusive storytelling.

In practice, the author promotes an exchange of ideas in storytelling events, where attendees examine narrative and graphic drafts before their completion. This shared interpretation reinforces their involvement and allows them to adjust the story, so the final version is a true and accurate portrayal of the message they want to convey. For instance, in a project that delves into the healthcare journeys of transgender people, the participants' comments pointed out nuances in expressions and phrasing that I had not considered; modifying those parts secured the quality of the final story (Streed et al., 2023).

Furthermore, reflexive meetings with the research team often serve as critical junctures where methodological insights and participant feedback converge to shape collective storytelling processes. Whether through iterative data workshops or community advisory meetings, these forums are invaluable for reviewing and interpreting narratives that challenge prevailing assumptions and foreground marginalized voices. Inclusive storytelling is both a methodological and an ethical exercise. Through respectful conversation, recognition of the socio-political context of participant stories, and use of multiple media for dissemination, researchers can empower participants and create new avenues for social transformation. Therefore, the dynamism of narrative inquiry converts static data into living stories that resonate across cultural and identity borders.

Closing

Designing and conducting inclusive research is a dynamic and reflexive process that demands awareness of diversity, commitment to methodological flexibility, and a steadfast dedication to ethical practice (Ralston, 2023). This chapter has outlined the fundamental elements required to build a research framework that honors diverse voices, from addressing the complexities of gender, religion, and socioeconomic status in research design to employing culturally competent data collection strategies and engaging in reflexive data interpretation. Experiences through the author's career have provided the realization that every stage of the research process—from recruitment and data collection to data analysis and writing of narratives—has to be settled through constant negotiations so as to enrich the participation of marginalized subjects. Here approaches, such as engagement with community partners, flexible interviewing possibilities for trans persons, and participatory storytelling to make narratives more inclusive, are moral imperatives as well as deepening and broadening the research findings (Divan et al., 2016). As one proceeds with data analyses, a critical examination through reflexivity is a blessing in disguise because one strives to guarantee that insights, interpretations, and conclusions foreground the participants' perspectives, for the researcher may be laden with biases. This means entering into partnership processes and engaging in constructive dialogues with community specialists as such practices foster deeper understandings and cultivate an inclusive and transformational research climate. An appeal to all researchers is to commit to inclusivity by adopting protocols that respect every cultural background and experience. This appeal is much more than a research procedure; it is an ethical obligation to nurture research communities that view diversity as a foundational pillar of academic creativity and equity. Truly inclusive approaches to research bring about deeper understanding, equalize knowledge creation processes, and elevate the voices of communities that have been marginalized within educational debates. In conclusion, the blueprint presented here is a practical guide for designing adaptive, respectful, and rigorously inclusive research. It is incumbent upon researchers to continue developing, refining, and sharing strategies that dissolve hierarchical structures within research processes so that every voice, regardless of gender, religion, socioeconomic background, or other identity markers, can contribute to meaningful and socially transformative research (DuBois et al., 2021; Ralston, 2023).

By integrating participatory research approaches, reflexivity, and culturally sensitive strategies into every phase of research, we may move together in creating an inclusive and representative social science agenda that respects and enriches the collected lived experience. One can understand that inclusive research strengthens scientific legitimacy, values personal histories and cultural identities central to social investigation, thereby carving a pathway for research to be considered ethical and innovative (Ralston, 2023). Here, the author urges all researchers to reflect on their practice, get ongoing feedback from various communities, and be willing to change methodologies to establish research spaces where all individuals are encouraged to co-produce knowledge, turning research into a tool of social transformation. It is believed that inclusive research methods can help bridge the gap between disconnected cultural groups and academic institutions, using sensitive data collection, critical interpretation, and respectful narration. This paradigm is a reminder to relentlessly advocate for equity, diversity, and social justice as core principles in research that, if truly implemented, can transform the academic world and deepen the collective grasp of humanity as a networked multi-layered phenomenon (Abramovich & Cleverley, 2018; Ralston, 2023; Walia & Mondal, 2025).

References

Abramovich, A., & Cleverley, K. (2018). A call to action: The urgent need for trans inclusive measures in mental health research. *The Canadian Journal of Psychiatry, 63*(8), 532–537.

Braybrook, D., Bristowe, K., Timmins, L., Roach, A., Day, E., Clift, P., Rose, R., Marshall, S., Johnson, K., Sleeman, K. E., & Harding, R. (2023). Communication about sexual orientation and gender between clinicians, LGBT+ people facing serious illness and their significant others: A qualitative interview study of experiences, preferences and recommendations. *BMJ Quality & Safety, 32*(2), 109–120. https://doi.org/10.1136/bmjqs-2022-014792

Cottrell, S. (2023). *Critical thinking skills* (4th ed.). Bloomsbury.

Divan, V., Cortez, C., Smelyanskaya, M., & Keatley, J. (2016). Transgender social inclusion and equality: A pivotal path to development. *Journal of the International AIDS Society, 19*, 20803.

DuBois, L. Z., Gibb, J. K., Juster, R. P., & Powers, S. I. (2021). Biocultural approaches to transgender and gender diverse experience and health: Integrating biomarkers and advancing gender/sex research. *American Journal of Human Biology, 33*(1), e23555.

Elischberger, H. B., Glazier, J. J., Hill, E. D., & Verduzco-Baker, L. (2018). Attitudes toward and beliefs about transgender youth: A cross-cultural comparison between the United States and India. *Sex roles, 78*(1), 142–160.

Forber-Pratt, A. J. (2024). Advancing and expecting inclusive research. *Inclusion, 12*(1), 30–39.

Miles, M. B., & Huberman, A. M. (1994). *Qualitative data analysis: An expanded sourcebook*. Sage.

Moolchaem, P., Liamputtong, P., O'Halloran, P., & Muhamad, R. (2015). The lived experiences of transgender persons: A meta-synthesis. *Journal of Gay & Lesbian Social Services, 27*(2), 143–171.

Nizza, I. E., Farr, J., & Smith, J. A. (2021). Achieving excellence in interpretative phenomenological analysis (IPA): Four markers of high quality. *Qualitative Research in Psychology, 18*(3), 369–386.

Ralston, A. L. (2023). *Is our research inclusive? Experiences in psychological research for participants identifying as transgender and gender diverse*. The University of Nebraska-Lincoln.

Rosenberg, S., & Tilley, P. M. (2021). 'A point of reference': The insider/outsider research staircase and transgender people's experiences of participating in trans-led research. *Qualitative Research, 21*(6), 923–938.

Singh, A. A., Richmond, K., & Burnes, T. R. (2013). Feminist participatory action research with transgender communities: Fostering the practice of ethical and empowering research designs. *International Journal of Transgenderism, 14*(3), 93–104.

Smith, J. A. (2011). Evaluating the contribution of interpretative phenomenological analysis. *Health Psychology Review, 5*(1), 9–27.

Smith, J. A. (2017). Interpretative phenomenological analysis: Getting at lived experience. *The Journal of Positive Psychology, 12*(3), 303–304.

Streed, C. G., Jr., Perlson, J. E., Abrams, M. P., & Lett, E. (2023). On, with, by—Advancing transgender health research and clinical practice. *Health Equity, 7*(1), 161–165.

Thomas, R., Pega, F., Khosla, R., Verster, A., Hana, T., & Say, L. (2017). Ensuring an inclusive global health agenda for transgender people. *Bulletin of the World Health Organization, 95*(2), 154.

Walia, S., & Mondal, S. (2025). Envisioning transgender equity: Amplifying global south narratives through inclusive archives and education. *Journal of International Women's Studies, 27*(3), 1–41.

5

Impact, Growth, and Reflection

Abstract For this pivot project, the experimentation with writing and expression of experience has a final chapter. This concluding chapter reflects on the author's evolution as a scholar-activist dedicated to transgender inclusivity. It explores the translation of academic research into tangible impact through scholarly communication, conference presentations, and strategic advocacy aimed at influencing policy and public perception. The narrative reflects on personal growth, key transformative moments, and the evolving perspectives on the responsibilities of a researcher. Expressing gratitude to mentors and communities, the chapter acknowledges the profound responsibility to inspire future generations. It concludes with a hopeful vision for the future of transgender rights in India and a powerful call to action for the academic community to embrace engaged, empathetic, and impactful research that serves the goal of social justice.

Keywords Scholar-activism • Knowledge translation • Research impact • Policy advocacy • Public scholarship • Personal transformation • Mentorship • Social justice • Academic responsibility

H. Kaur, *Psychological Research Among Transgender Individuals*,
https://doi.org/10.1007/978-3-032-12051-9_5

The author is a scholar-activist committed to discussing the academic narratives and building academic spaces affirming transgender identities. Her experiences with the community and her critical research continuously uplift one another, each shaping the other. On the same lines her identity is built on a strong commitment to unspooling normative presumptions. Her work seeks to braid into a conceptual framework for academic exploration, community engagement, and policy activism to drive transformation in education and institutional contexts. This chapter discusses how she supports transgender inclusion through several channels, such as rigorous scholarly authorship, participatory involvement in academic conferences, and strategic means of implementing research findings into applicable policy change.

Advocating through Scholarship

The research is based on a fundamentally ethically pluralistic perspective; therefore, it values trans voices and resists deep-rooted normative paradigms. The author has intentionally built research programs that adopt participatory methodology to enable transgender communities to emerge as co-producers of knowledge and not just as research subjects. This approach is critical to genuine and respectful inquiry. The writer has aimed at making their writing clear, expressive, and readable, continually striving to use language that respects the different identities along the transgender spectrum and refrains from reductive and pathologizing descriptions. The research became a part of is built upon an in-built ethically pluralistic perspective; therefore, it gives precedence to trans voices and subverts entrenched normative paradigms. She has specifically structured research programs with inclusive participatory methodology so that transgender populations can become co-producers of knowledge instead of objects of study. It is a required approach for respectful and valid inquiry.

The author has endeavored to make her own writing understandable, readable, and accessible, always attempting to employ language that is respectful of the differing identities along the transgender spectrum and does not make reductive or pathologizing descriptions. For instance, in any conference presentation, one can narrate transgender students' lived experiences in the sciences while providing an empirical counternarrative to the standard deficit models that attempt to portray them solely through tales of resilience and systemic impediments.

The peer-reviewed publications and the critical reviews they have incurred show that academic writing can be rigorous and even deeply transformative when centered on genuine transgender stories and disrupting systemic frameworks. The author used theoretical frameworks like intersectionality, ecological systems theory, and transgender theory to undergird her analyses and to bring to the fore the complexity of transgender identity in scholarly discourse. She has also delivered addresses at trans-inclusive symposiums where she shared research findings with diverse audiences of academics, educators, and community leaders, reinforcing the importance of bridging theoretical insight with real-world application. Moreover, the authors' academic work includes a variety of formats, from peer-reviewed articles to edited volumes in which she meticulously documents the multifaceted dimensions of transgender experiences across social, educational, and policy contexts. More specifically, she has worked on writing projects that challenge conventional identity development models and promote more fluid, non-linear models that better reflect transgender lives, as witnessed through her work in academic journals and edited collections. Furthermore, her work focuses on the power of scholarship to transform when it intentionally considers institutional power dynamics and translates those analyses into actionable suggestions for change. More specifically, she has worked on writing projects that challenge conventional models of identity development and promote more fluid, non-linear models that better reflect transgender lives, as witnessed through her work in academic journals and edited collections. Furthermore, her work highlights the power of scholarship to transform when it intentionally considers institutional power dynamics and translates those analyses into actionable suggestions for change.

She has also explicitly reflected on her positionality as both an insider and an outsider, an act which challenges existing epistemologies and encourages a critical self-awareness that enriches the overall inclusivity of her work. The need for direct, clear communication in scholarship cannot be overemphasized. Through accessible language, the author has extended her reach to wide-ranging constituencies, ranging from academic colleagues to policymakers, ensuring that her research is heard beyond academia.

From Research to Action

One of the main ideas of a scholar-activist approach is that scholars try to give advocacy a tangible, pragmatic aspect. She has thus devoted herself to ensuring that insight gained from academic inquiry leads to policy changes and community empowerment, and she encourages all her readers to consider it. To understand it better, an example can be given: research on transgender youth in education can enter into legislative debate on the issue of school safety policies by informing lawmakers of the urgent need to create inclusive processes aimed at protecting vulnerable communities. The interdisciplinary collaborations have also involved working alongside community organizations and advocacy groups to jointly develop research findings into specific policy recommendations to address some pressing issues facing institutions today. One critical successful intervention was the joint effort with local advocates to develop and implement a new campus policy concerning the use of preferred names and pronouns in university administrative systems, so much so that the changes have given transgender students a vastly improved experience in their day-to-day lives.

Complementing this success was her involvement in policy roundtables, where she contributed background statistics on the systemic barriers experienced by transgender persons that aided in turning academic knowledge into instruments for advocacy and legal reform. In addition, she has joined with community-based outreach organizations to create workshops and training sessions for educators and administrators that nurture an awareness and active engagement regarding transgender inclusivity. Her attempt to bridge the gulf-cutting applied practice between theoretical research and practice further strengthens the notion that scholarly endeavors must go beyond writing across the aisles and into the direct engagement of policy debates and community initiatives again, something which several of her successful collaborations reaffirm.

However, such translation efforts come with challenges: the continued disjunction between academic discourse and the policymaking environment is often the matter to be negotiated through extended relationship-building across stakeholders. While these obstacles exist, the payoff of seeing real change materialize, like enhanced mental health services for transgender youths, is a testament to the effectiveness of these advocacy efforts. She then discovered that research-writer-translation-for-policy is a constantly changing process in which one must translate empirical evidence into plain language without weakening the rigor of our process.

She has always been motivated by the belief that if strategically allied with community expertise and policy advocacy, academic research could be used for dismantling oppressive structures and affecting real change. Having experienced some of these processes taking steps of their own toward new research collaborations, currently investigating institutional doctrines and instigating updated policies with concrete impacts on the lives of the transgender communities, is a good acknowledgment of that. Her projects, with an awareness of purpose and social responsibility, link scholarship and functional outcomes to change institutional cultures.

Growth and Transformation

The scholar-activist pathway is one of growth, reflection, and transformation, with professional breakthroughs and personal revelations. Initially, in the baby steps of her research, she encountered an awareness of the limitations posed by the conventional gender binary framework. Thus, it was increasingly apparent that we should develop and apply more complicated and intersectional frameworks for academic credibility and true social justice. She remembers crucial moments in those early commitments of my works to paper and to the stage and audience at academic conferences, when remarks on transgender inclusivity from myriad directions only fueled my commitment to resolve the divide between theory and lived experience. Over time, interactions with transgender community members, who shared their personal struggles with institutional discrimination and misrepresentation, profoundly influenced my perspective and encouraged her to reframe my research questions to address the real needs of these communities better.

In an absolutely transformative evolution of my academic orientation, there is a shift from a peripheral interest view to a leading stage site for social justice, equal representation, and human dignity. In such development, she studied the professional development of rigorous self-reflections that interrogated my privileges and limits to research. This inquiry elevated the scholarship and my practice of mentorship so that emerging scholars must be counseled through their journey toward inclusive scholarship. In the scholarly debates and during mentorship with various scholars, she has learned that transformation is an endless process available for critique, renouncing past-held assumptions, and fostering sustained learning. A few major turning points in my intellectual evolution include recognizing the gap between normative research practices and the lived realities of transgender people, which motivated me to embrace methodological approaches that honor lived experience and foster ethical collaboration.

Reflecting on these experiences, one realizes that their work and personal growth have mutually reinforced each other. Challenges have fostered slow change in one's academic courses and my commitment to social justice. Different perspectives created innovative ways of blending intersectional perspectives with empirical research. Hence, one becomes an advocate who champions the rights and dignity of trans persons in my very own life construction. This learning-filled journey and the development of her own identity affirm that academic activism is both a personal and collective endeavor. Therefore, this movement must keep reconstructing itself by valuing change and transformation. Researchers enjoy the delicate dance of research, community input, and self-creation. Here, she remains committed to ushering in the call for scholarship-oriented work as much toward healing and empowerment as it is toward intellectual rigor. Reflection on specific moments of vulnerability, resilience, and triumph illustrates that my journeys in academia and activism are bound so tightly that it is from this understanding that one can illicitly shape the shape of her work. Furthermore, collaborative engagements with scholars and community groups have provided me with fresh insights and reinforced an enduring sense of purpose and solidarity.

Gratitude and Responsibility

The author has always been very grateful for those mentors, colleagues, and transgender communities who would remain by her side, supporting , giving honest feedback, and sharing a mutual commitment toward justice. The intellectual mentoring she received from highly established scholars in the field of transgender studies, in addition to the community advocates' hands-on instruction, was key to shaping her methodological and theoretical leanings. The author acknowledges that such learnings in this field cannot be attributed solely to her but rather that it was made possible by the generosity of those who shared their biographies, knowledge, and often quite incisive insights to help her steer through the tricky waters of normative structures and build an academic discourse that is just a bit more inclusive.

Throughout every project handled together, from journal articles to policy workshops and beyond, the author recognizes that collaborative knowledge production and political action are founded on their shared responsibility to create room for those voices that remain marginalized. This shared responsibility urges her to mentor budding researchers and activist scholars through processes of methodological transparency and ethical rigor in their research. Here, urging emerging scholar-activists to remain steadfast in their commitment to integrating lived experiences into academic inquiry, even when any pressures or backlash threaten to derail their efforts. The journey shows one that true scholarly advocacy remains differentiated in intellectual curiosity versus tenacious social justice. At the same time, advising emerging academics to consider that every research project, conference presentation, or policy engagement is part of some larger movement aiming at change. Sincerely thanking the academic and activist communities that continuously challenge the status quo and constantly remind us that we must engage in intersectional and inclusive approaches in all realms of research and policy.

Nurtured by a synergistic reciprocal relationship, mutual empowerment, and shared visions of societal transformation lies the foundational line voiding the collective burden that is set to offer future generations of researchers and activists. Lastly, the author reminds herself and others:

cultivating an ethos of gratitude and accountability is worthwhile to keep the quest for long-haul advocacy alive; crucially, this mindset preserves our attainment from ever becoming a form of an endpoint toward which we rest and turn with little intention but as the stepping stone for more bold and mind-bending endeavors.

Any researcher's commitment to transgender inclusivity is a personal ethic and academic imperative that fuels their research and advocacy. The vision for a just and equitable society. The synergy of rigorous scholarship, participation in conferences, and intentional translation of research into policy work enables the otherwise perplexing world of the cisnormative to curl into a manageable set of concrete programmatic choices. In each scholarly engagement, be it publishing a reflective article, engaging in tough debates during academic conferences, or working with co-stakeholders from communities, a thread is being stitched into the larger realm of transformation.

The author hardly dares to depart from this hope and, with complete conviction, invites readers, colleagues, along with generations of scholar-activists yet to come, to join each other in this endeavor, as transforming academia and society remains an ongoing work. Until we have remade every fiber threaded with marginality into a domain of justice, the struggle must not rest. May this chapter be a testimony to our past efforts and a thick layer of dust on any shelving, so warmly totes a clarion call for future action, that ought to tap away at our consciousness, celebrating what we have accomplished yet remaining fully awake and ever diligent about the work of gender inclusivity in the trans discourse. An invitation to amplify voices the majority had intended silencing; to heed this call, contribute toward altering the pathway of destiny by telling your stories, cracking down on barriers that restrain, and envisioning a liberated world of equity, respect, and belonging for everyone in unison. Rallying for trans justice embodies the spirit of human solidarity. It lays the foundation for hope and justice for that future where dignity is awarded to every identity and a community is forged for every person. Though it may seem daunting, the stakes of reimagining this world are far higher, and the onus of transforming all these myriad hands into concrete changes for the generations yet unborn rests on all of us.

Concluding Comments

For many of us, the Navtej Singh Johar judgment of 2018 is converting a much-cited moment into the locus of attention in the history of LGBTQ+ rights in India. Symbolically, it did away with one period replete with colonial oppression and heralded another based on dignity and constitutional rights. The decision was praised as a strong celebration of privacy, individual freedom, and the humanity of queer people, notably from the urban, middle-class, and elite strata of society who had some level of legal access and advocacy. However, as much as this ruling had symbolic weight, the focus on privacy and decriminalization offered insufficient attention to other critical aspects. By focusing mainly on the right to engage in consensual acts in private spaces, it left many broader issues of structural inequality, public recognition, and everyday discrimination unaddressed. As one scholar, Mehta (2021), indicates, such progress, while historic, tends to present queer rights in terms of individual freedom inside the closet, a step that is needed, though not the culmination of the battle for complete social and legal equality.

Every scene of social justice seems to fly upward as further-chained-down systemic inequalities. Legal improvements have failed to address the deep-rooted economic disenfranchisement that plagues the lives of many LGBT populations, especially those of marginalized groups: the working-class, Dalits, and transgender individuals. For this particular group of people, it is like an assurance let out on the symbolic weight of decriminalizing Section 377. However, they do not survive with legal protection against socioeconomic discrimination, day-to-day violence, or harassment at the hands of police (Srivastava & Kumar, 2019). The realization of constitutional entitlements varies enormously among communities of gay men in everyday life; the symbolic reasoning of constitutional victories conceals these variations. Researchers and anthropologists have shown that real material conditions often negate the potential for legal change (Mehta, 2021). Due to systemic barriers and deep-rooted prejudices within their communities and the lack of institutional support, these transgender individuals still face systemic barriers to accessing healthcare, education, and employment (Arvind et al., 2022; Chakrapani et al., 2023). As a result, the legal narratives that come from elite judicial and policy discourses stand in sharp contrast to the lived realities of many people who identify as LGBT.

A question arises: are Indian transgender persons happy to be clustered in LGBTQIA+, or do their experiences vary because they are not sexual minorities but are gender minorities? Maybe for our ease, we categorized them, but should this knowledge be required to be reconstructed? Leaving you with these thoughts!!!

References

Arvind, A., Pandya, A., Amin, L., Aggarwal, M., Agrawal, D., Tiwari, K., et al. (2022). Social strain, distress, and gender dysphoria among transgender women and Hijra in Vadodara, India. *International Journal of Transgender Health, 23*(1–2), 149–163.

Chakrapani, V., Newman, P. A., Shunmugam, M., Rawat, S., Mohan, B. R., Baruah, D., & Tepjan, S. (2023). A scoping review of lesbian, gay, bisexual, transgender, queer, and intersex (LGBTQI+) people's health in India. *PLOS Global Public Health, 3*(4), e0001362.

Mehta, J. (2021). An Interesting Journey of an LGBTQ Professional. *NHRD Network Journal, 14*(3), 346–349. https://doi.org/10.1177/26314541211030591 (Original work published 2021)

Srivastava, A., & Kumar, V. (2019). Section 377 and LGBT activism in India. *International Journal of Research and Analytical Reviews, 6*(2), 30–4.

Appendices

Research Tools and Resources forUnderstanding Transgender Inclusive Research

Guidelines and Frameworks

- UNESCO Inclusive Policy Lab Toolkit—Guidance on inclusive policy research and participatory methods.
- https://en.unesco.org/inclusivepolicylab/e-teams/inclusive-and-participatory-youth-policy-southeast-asia/documents
- American Psychological Association (APA) Guidelines on Inclusive Language—Practical recommendations for avoiding bias in language use.https://www.apa.org/about/apa/equity-diversity-inclusion/language-guide.pdf
- National Institutes of Health (NIH) Inclusion Policy—Standards for the inclusion of diverse populations in research.
- https://grants.nih.gov/policy-and-compliance/policy-topics/inclusion

H. Kaur, *Psychological Research Among Transgender Individuals*,
https://doi.org/10.1007/978-3-032-12051-9

- Transgender persons act https://www.indiacode.nic.in/bitstream/123456789/13091/1/a2019-40.pdf
- Mental Health Act, 2017 https://www.indiacode.nic.in/bitstream/123456789/2249/1/A2017-10.pdf
- Ministry of Social Justice and Empowerment, Government of India: https://socialjustice.gov.in/
- Ministry of health and welfare: https://mohfw.gov.in/
- Ministry of Education, National Education Policy 2020:
- NISD: https://www.nisd.gov.in/
- Framework by GATE: Global NGO for Trans Equality: https://gate.ngo/
- UN-SDG: SDG 3: https://sdgs.un.org/goals/goal3

Software and Platforms

1. Dedoose—Qualitative and mixed-methods analysis software with tools for demographic segmentation. https://www.dedoose.com/
2. ATLAS.ti- helps researchers analyze unstructured data, making it easier to capture and understand themes like identity, marginalization, and lived experiences in inclusive research. http://ATLAS.ti
3. NVivo—Supports analysis of diverse participant perspectives; includes coding schemes for inclusivity. https://lumivero.com/products/nvivo/
4. Qualtrics—Customizable demographic questions that allow for non-binary and culturally sensitive options. https://www.qualtrics.com/en-au/free-account/
5. For understanding world level mapping for transgender persons as per laws and policies: https://ilga.org/ilga-world-maps/

Training Resources

6. National Center for Faculty Development & Diversity—Workshops on inclusive research practices. https://academicaffairs.ucdavis.edu/ncfdd

7. Coursera: Diversity & Inclusion in Research—Modules on ethical and methodological considerations for marginalized groups. https://www.coursera.org/campus?utm_content=corp-to-landing-for-campus&utm_campaign=website&utm_medium=coursera&utm_source=header&utm_term=b-out
8. GATE Toolkit: The Politics is Trans Toolkit is a collection of two interconnected resources designed to empower trans and gender-diverse people to participate in politics and advocate for systemic change. https://gate.ngo/wp-content/uploads/2025/05/Politics-is-Trans_Guide_English.pdf
9. Center for Research on Gender and Sexuality—Academic training materials and case studies. https://gendersexuality.uchicago.edu/
10. PGPR: For readers seeking additional support with the presentation of qualitative research, the team at Post Graduate Proof Reader (PGPR), led by Johanna Spiers, offers professional proofreading and feedback services. Their work is particularly focused on social science disciplines and the team have expertise in interpretative phenomenological analysis (IPA) and other qualitative approaches. Details of their services and team can be found on their website: https://www.postgradproofreader.co.uk/
11. **TAPAS:** Training for augmenting productivity and services by NISD, Basic course on transgender issues can be accessed at: https://tapas.dosje.gov.in/ilms/

Sample Interview Protocols for Working with Transgender Participants

Pre-Interview Preparation

1. Review inclusive language guidelines (avoid misgendering; ask pronouns at start).
2. Ensure interview space (physical or virtual) is private, safe, and affirming.

3. Provide consent forms that include participants' preferred names and pronouns.
4. Offer the choice to skip any question without penalty.
5. Respect their time and preferences for the interview.

Sample Opening Script

"Thank you for agreeing to participate. Before we start, I want to confirm your name and pronouns so I can address you correctly throughout. You can decline to answer any question at any time. Everything we discuss will be kept confidential unless you choose otherwise. Do you have any questions before we begin?"

Exemplars

6. Can you share your personal journey and experiences with genderidentity?
7. How have social, institutional, or community contexts impacted your daily life?

Probe: How do you think society impacts your daily life? Probe: How does your community impact your life?

Probe: How do people who are not trans impact your lives?

8. What resources or supports have been most meaningful to you?
9. What challenges have you faced in healthcare, education, or workplace environments?
10. Is there anything you wish researchers better understood about transgender experiences?

Closing Script

"Thank you for sharing your time and experiences. Your voice is an important part of this work. If you'd like, we can send you a copy of the findings. Here's information on support services if you need them."

Index[1]

[1] Note: Page numbers followed by 'n' refer to notes.

H. Kaur, *Psychological Research Among Transgender Individuals*,
https://doi.org/10.1007/978-3-032-12051-9

FSC
www.fsc.org
MIX
Papier | Fördert gute Waldnutzung
FSC® C083411

Kolibri 360 GmbH
Ferdinand-Jühlke-Straße 7
99095 Erfurt, Deutschland
produktsicherheit@kolibri360.de